For more information...

The following free booklets may be helpful if your loved one has cancer treatment:

- *Chemotherapy and You*

- *Coping With Advanced Cancer*

- *Eating Hints for Cancer Patients*

- *Taking Part in Cancer Treatment Research Studies*

- *Pain Control*

- *Radiation Therapy and You*

- *Taking Time*

- *Thinking About Complementary and Alternative Medicine*

- *When Cancer Returns*

These booklets are available from the National Cancer Institute (NCI). To learn more about specific types of cancer or to request any of these booklets, visit NCI's website (http://www.cancer.gov). You can also call NCI's Cancer Information Service toll-free at 1-800-4-CANCER (1-800-422-6237) to speak with an information specialist.

We would like to offer our sincerest gratitude to the extraordinary caregivers, health professionals, and scientists who contributed to the development and review of this publication.

When Someone You Love
Has Advanced Cancer

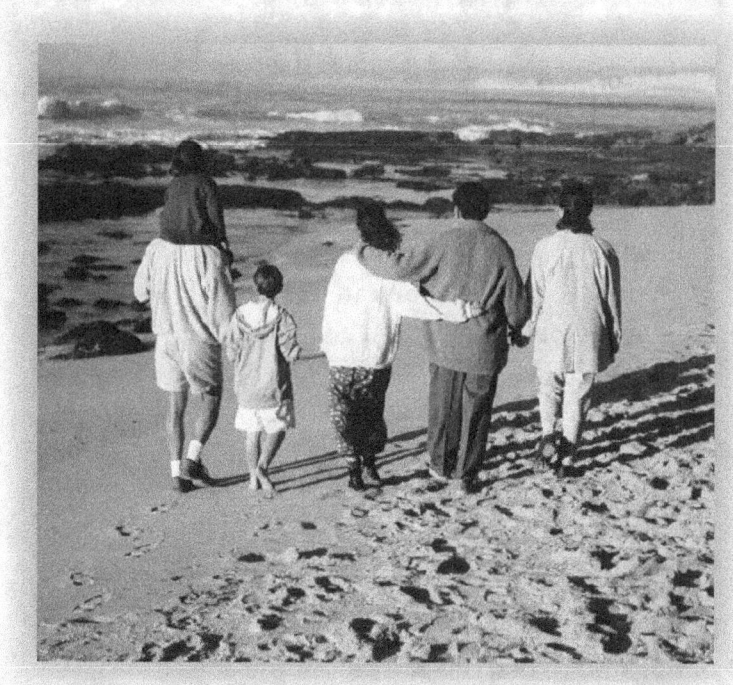

"If there's one thing
that's come out of taking care of someone,
it's that I've learned what's important
really fast. And it's a lesson
I'll carry forever."
—Maureen

The purpose of this book is to focus on *you* and *your needs*.

We've heard from many caregivers about things they wish they had known early on. We have collected their tips in this booklet. Some of the tips seem simple, but they may not always be easy to do.

Use this booklet in whatever way works best for you. You can read it from front to back. Or you can just refer to different sections as you need them.

No two people are alike. Some chapters of this booklet may apply to you, while others may not. Or you may find that some sections are more useful to you later. Or you may decide that you would rather read a different booklet right now (see below).

Terms Used: This booklet uses the terms **"loved one"** and **"patient"** throughout to describe the person you are caring for. In addition, for ease of reading, we alternate using the pronouns **"he"** and **"she"** when referring to the person with cancer.

Other booklets for caregivers that can be ordered or printed from the NCI website are:

- *Facing Forward: When Someone You Love Has Completed Cancer Treatment*

- *When Someone You Love Is Being Treated for Cancer*

- *Young People With Cancer: A Handbook for Parents*

- *When Your Parent Has Cancer: A Guide For Teens*

- *When Your Brother or Sister Has Cancer: A Guide for Teens*

Table of Contents

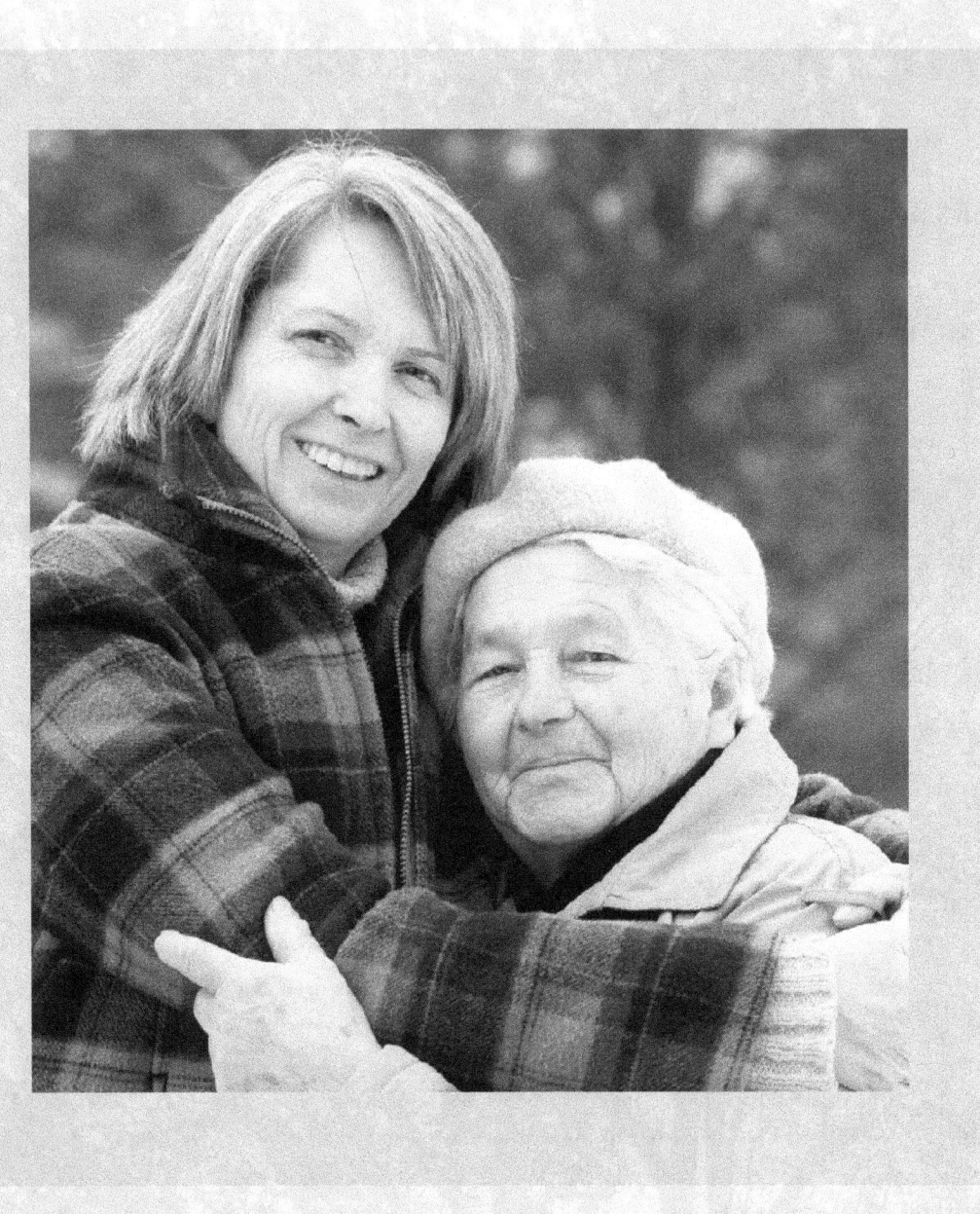

Is This Booklet for Me?

This booklet is for you if your loved one has been told that he or she has advanced cancer that is no longer responding to treatment. It explores many of the questions and crossroads you may be facing now.

Until now, you have probably gone through cancer treatment with your loved one hoping for a remission or recovery. If your health care team is telling you that this may not be possible, you may be facing new choices to make about care and future steps.

There are other booklets available that talk about how to give care to a loved one. But the purpose of this booklet is to focus on you and your needs.

Making these transitions in care can be hard. You'll need to focus on the things you can control and what you can do to make this time with your loved one special. You'll want to help the patient live life to the fullest. Many caregivers say that this time gave their life special meaning and a sense of what's important.

Who Is a Caregiver?

If you are helping someone you love during cancer care, you are a "caregiver." You may not think of yourself as a caregiver. You may look at what you're doing as something natural—taking care of someone you love.

There are different types of caregivers. Some are family members. Others are friends. Every situation is different. So there are different ways to give care. There isn't one way that works best.

Caregiving can mean helping with day-to-day activities such as doctor visits or preparing food. But it can also happen long-distance, when you are coordinating care and services by phone or email. Caregiving can also mean giving emotional and spiritual support. You may be helping your loved one cope and work through the many feelings that come up at this time. Talking, listening, and just being there are some of the most important things you can do.

During this time, the natural r esponse of most caregivers is to put their own feelings and needs aside. They try to focus on the person with cancer and the many tasks of caregiving. This may be fine for a little while. But it can be hard to keep up for a long time. And it's not good for your health. If you don't take care of yourself, you won't be able to take care of others. It's important for everyone that you take care of *you*.

Helping Your Loved One Cope With Advanced Cancer

"When you're taking care of somebody, you're so busy. For me, staying busy was very fulfilling. But then, when it began to shift, I felt empty sometimes, wondering what to do next." —Joe

Your loved one may be struggling with advanced cancer or with a cancer recurrence. Doctors may be saying that the cancer isn't responding to treatment. You may have been told that long-term remission isn't likely. Or your loved one may have decided to discontinue treatment and live out his or her days to the fullest.

This may be a time when new decisions need to be made. Shifts in care may be needed or may already be taking place. The burden of making these decisions together may seem much heavier than it used to be. These choices often come with many emotions, such as sadness, anger, and the fear of the unknown. They may also come with questions about how much longer your loved one will live.

Thinking or talking about these issues may feel like you're giving up. But you aren't. It doesn't mean giving up hope. People usually cope better when they have different options. Having information about how to deal with tough situations will help. Your loved one still deserves good medical care and support from the health care team even if the treatment changes.

Making Decisions Together

You may have been caring for the cancer patient for a short or a long time. Most likely, you'll be very involved in helping make choices about next steps for care. Some of these choices may include:

- Treatment goals
- When to use hospice care
- Financial decisions
- How to get support from family members

"I guess some people don't want a lot of information because they aren't sure they can handle what the possibilities are. But I don't think you can really make a good decision without knowing everything. We had to ask a lot of questions, though, because we didn't know all our options." —Beth

When dealing with advanced cancer, people have different goals for their care. Some want to keep following more aggressive treatments. Others decide to choose other paths for care. You may wonder: "Have we done everything possible to treat the cancer, or should we try another treatment?" It's natural to want to do all you can, but you should weigh these feelings against the positives and negatives for your loved one.

Questions to ask:

- What's the best we can hope for by trying another treatment?

- Is this treatment meant to ease side effects or slow the spread of cancer?

- Is there a chance that a new treatment will be found while we try the old one?

- What are the possible side effects and other downsides of the treatment? How likely are they?

- Are the possible rewards bigger than the possible drawbacks?

"You really want to know if the treatment is worse than the illness. We've come to ask the question, what's the quality of life after this? Is it worth being sick for 2 months if he's got less than a year to live?" —Dan

Asking these questions may help the patient decide whether to continue or begin more treatment. It's best to work together on this process. It will help you figure out both of your needs and the needs of others close to you.

It's important to ask your health care team what to expect in the future. And it's also important to be clear with them about how much information you and the patient want from them.

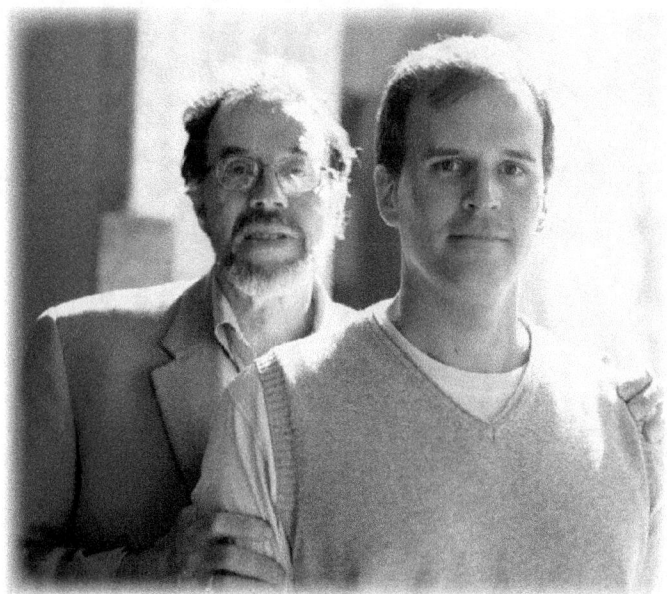

Understanding Your Loved One's Wishes

For many families, it's important that your loved one be in charge of making decisions. But in some families and cultures, it's common for the caregiver to make many of the decisions. And they may make them with or without the patient knowing. Or sometimes the patient wants the caregiver to make all the decisions. This may be hard, for many reasons:

- Your own stress may make it hard to decide.

- Your ideas about how to move forward may differ from the ideas of other family members or friends.

- The patient may have different beliefs about care than you or other loved ones.

- The opinions of your health care team may differ from your loved one's or yours.

"I think some people, like me, want to know everything. I want no surprises. But my husband doesn't want to know anything. We struggle with how to handle this issue."
—Dora

There may also come a time when you have to make decisions for your loved one because he can't anymore. It's important to get a sense of how he feels about this before it happens. How would he like to deal with it? This may mean letting go of some opinions that you have about treatment. (For example, you may want to keep your loved one alive, whatever it takes. But he may wish to stop receiving life-sustaining measures at a certain point.) Try to keep things in perspective by looking at the facts.

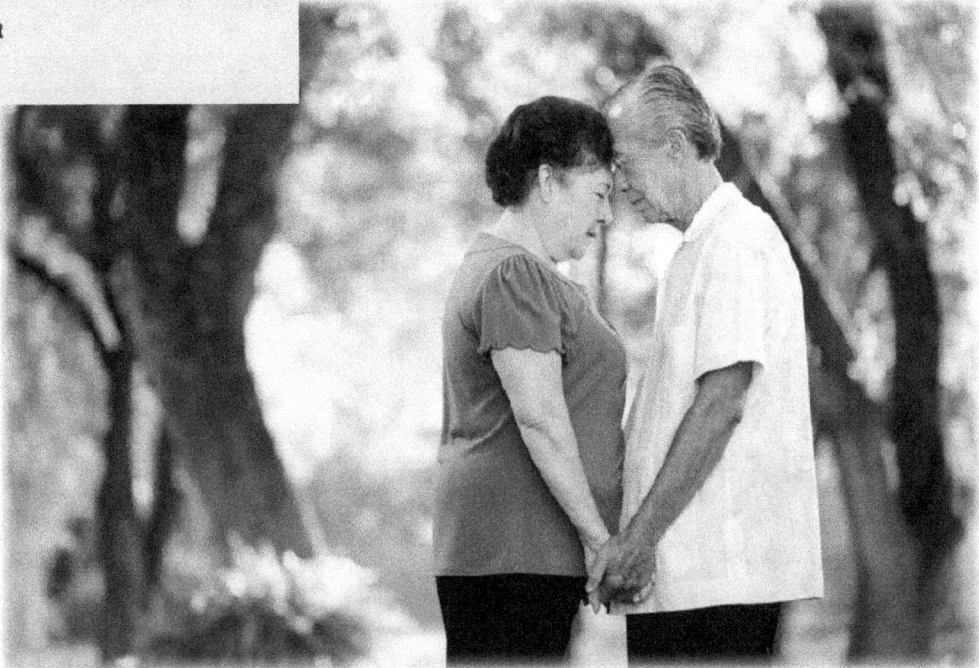

Palliative Care

All patients have a right to comfort and quality of life throughout their care. Care that makes patients feel better, but doesn't treat the disease itself is often called **palliative care**. It includes treating or preventing cancer symptoms and side effects caused by treatment. Comfort care can also mean getting help with emotional and spiritual problems during and after cancer treatment.

> Sometimes patients only want to focus on the cancer itself. Yet they can improve their quality of life with palliative care.

People once thought of palliative care as a way to comfort those dying of cancer. Doctors now offer this care to all cancer patients, beginning when the cancer is diagnosed. Palliative care can go on through treatment, survival, advanced disease, and the time when treatment no longer controls the cancer. Members of the health care team may be able to provide comfort care. But a palliative care specialist may be the best person to treat some problems. Ask the doctor or nurse if there is a specialist your loved one can see.

Choices for Care

There are a number of options for your loved one's cancer care. These depend on the type of cancer and the patient's goals for care. These options include:

- Clinical trials (research studies)
- Palliative radiation, chemotherapy, or surgery
- Hospice care
- Home care

Many patients choose more than one option. Your loved one should base her decision on the risks and benefits of available treatments as well as her own feelings about life and death. You should both ask all the questions you need to. If she chooses *not* to get any more active cancer treatment, it does not necessarily mean a quick decline and death. And she will continue to receive palliative care and made comfortable. The health care team can offer information and advice on treatment options.

> "We have to let patients and their family members truly understand that if they choose not to do chemo or some other aggressive therapy, there are other options where they will receive support, comfort care, and assistance from the health care team." —Dr. Hauser

Clinical Trials

Clinical trials are research studies using people that try to find better ways to treat cancer. Every day, cancer researchers learn more about treatment options from clinical trials.

The trial your loved one may choose will depend on the type of cancer he has. It will also depend on what treatments he has already had. Each study has rules about who can take part. These rules may include the patient's age, health, and type of cancer.

Clinical trials have both benefits and risks. Your doctor and the study doctors should fully explain these before any decisions are made.

Taking part in a clinical trial could help your loved one, and also help others who get cancer in the future. But insurance and managed care plans do not always cover the costs. What they cover varies by plan and by study. Talk with your health care team to learn more about coverage for clinical trials.

For more information about clinical trials, see NCI's booklet, *Taking Part in Cancer Treatment Research Studies* (see inside cover).

Palliative Radiation, Chemotherapy, or Surgery

Some palliative radiation, chemotherapy, and surgeries may help relieve pain and other symptoms. In this way, they may improve a person's quality of life even if they don't slow the cancer. These treatments may be given to remove or shrink a tumor. Or they may be given to slow down a tumor's spread. For more information, see the NCI booklets, *Chemotherapy and You* and *Radiation Therapy and You* (see inside cover).

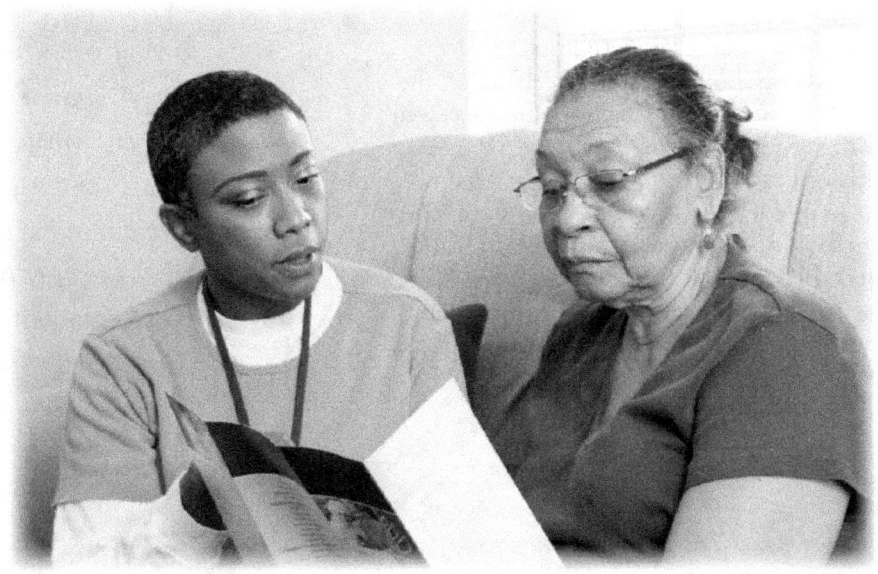

Hospice Care

Choosing hospice care doesn't mean that you've given up. It means that the treatment goals are different now. It does not mean giving up hope, but rather changing what you hope for.

The goal of hospice is to help patients live each day to the fullest by making them as comfortable and as symptom-free as possible. Hospice doctors, nurses, chaplains, social workers, and volunteers are specially trained. They are dedicated to supporting the emotional, social, and spiritual needs of both patients and their families, as well as dealing with patients' medical symptoms.

Many people believe that hospice is only available in the last days or weeks of life. They don't realize that hospice can provide support for much more than a few weeks. As a result, many caregivers have said that they wished they had gotten hospice involved sooner in the care process. They were surprised by the expert care and understanding that they got. Often, control of symptoms not only improves quality of life but also helps people live longer. Check with the hospice you are thinking of using to learn what treatments and services are covered. Also check with your loved one's insurance company to see what it will cover.

People usually qualify for hospice services when their doctor signs a statement that says that patients with their type and stage of disease, on average, aren't likely to survive beyond 6 months. Patients will be reviewed periodically by the health care team to see whether hospice care is still right for them. Services may include:

- Doctor services

- Nursing care

- Medical supplies and equipment

- Drugs for managing cancer-related symptoms and pain

- Short-term inpatient care

- Homemaker and home health aide services

- Respite services to give you a break from caring for your loved one

- Counseling

- Social work services

- Spiritual care

- Bereavement (grief) counseling and support

- Volunteer services

> "I can't say enough about our hospice nurse. We don't need her all the time yet, but she's here if we need help. She comes by or calls us to see if there's anything she can do. She's been a great source of comfort these past few months." —Gail

No One Knows the Future

It's normal for people to want to know how long their loved one will have to live. It's also natural to want to prepare for what lies ahead. You may want to prepare emotionally too, as well as make certain arrangements and plans.

But predicting how long someone will live is difficult. The doctor has to take into account the type of cancer, treatment, past illnesses, and other factors. Your loved one's doctor may be able to give you an estimate. But keep in mind that it's a guess. Every patient is different.

Some patients live long past the time the doctor first predicted. Others live a shorter time. Also, an infection or other complication could happen and change things. Your loved one's doctor may know the situation best. But even the doctor can't know the answer for sure. And doctors don't always feel comfortable trying to predict how long someone will live.

In truth, none of us knows when we are going to die. Unexpected events happen every day. The best we can do is try to live fully and for today.

What to Expect with Hospice Care

People can get hospice services at home, in special facilities, in hospitals, and in nursing homes. Hospice care also provides visits by nursing assistants, social workers, and chaplains, as well as nurses on call 24 hours a day in case you need advice. And they have many volunteers who help families care for their loved one. Some hospice services will give palliative chemotherapy at home as well. Hospice care doesn't seek to treat cancer. But it does treat curable problems with brief hospital stays if needed. Examples might be pneumonia or a bladder infection.

> "I wish I'd found out earlier about hospice care. But you don't know what you need at the beginning. And I didn't realize they could help me sooner, rather than later." —Bruce

Medicare, Medicaid, and most private insurance companies cover hospice services. For those without coverage and in financial need, many hospices provide care for free. To learn more about hospice care, call the National Hospice and Palliative Care Organization at 1-800-658-8898. Or visit the website at http://www.nhpco.org to find a hospice program in your community.

Home Care

Home care services not only provide palliative care, but may treat the cancer itself. This is for people who get medical care at home rather than in a hospital. If the patient qualifies for home care services, they may include:

- Managing symptoms
- Monitoring care
- Physical and other therapies
- Providing medical equipment

Your loved one may have to pay for home care services. Check with your insurance company. Medicare, Medicaid, and private insurance companies will sometimes cover home care services when ordered by the doctor. But some rules apply. So talk to a social worker and other members of the health care team to find out more about home care.

Working With the Health Care Team

Your situation may be changing a lot now. It's very important to keep asking questions. Some caregivers feel that they were given a lot of information early on, but not as much later. And learning all the unknowns of the different care and treatment options can be stressful.

It's important for you and your loved one to sit down with the health care team. You need to talk about future steps and what to expect. You may be afraid of what you might hear. But other caregivers have said that they felt reassured after learning their options. It made them able to plan ahead.

Some people with cancer want to know everything. Others let their caregivers make the decisions. Sometimes these differences are cultural. Other times they are personal. The patient, your family, and you should decide who will be the primary contact for the health care team.

Asking About Pain

People who have their pain managed are able to focus on enjoying life. Caregivers often worry about their loved one being in pain. If they are preoccupied by pain, you may notice changes in their personality, such as being distant, not being able to sleep, or not being able to focus on daily activities they once enjoyed.

Your loved one does not have to be in pain or in any discomfort. Some people assume that there will always be severe pain with cancer. This is not true. Pain can be managed throughout treatment. The key is to talk regularly with the health care team about pain and other symptoms. You may want to ask if there is a pain specialist on staff as well.

Sometimes people with cancer don't want to talk to the health care team about their pain. They worry that others will think that they're complaining or that pain means the cancer is getting worse. Or they think that pain is just something they have to accept. Sometimes people get so used to pain, they forget what it's like to live without it. The medical team should ask about pain levels, but it's up to *you and the patient* to be open about any pain she is having.

"It can be hard for me as a doctor, because many times I see patients who want to know everything. And then I have caregivers who **don't** want me to tell the patient everything. Yet the reality is that the patients know their bodies—they know what's going on. So sometimes I get a situation where everyone knows the truth but tries to keep it from the other person to protect them." —Dr. Crawford

Your Loved One's Eating

It's okay to offer your loved one food, but try not to pressure him to eat. We often think of eating well as bringing good health. But when people have advanced cancer, they may not have an appetite. Also, their bodies may need less food than in the past. Or, some people find it easier to eat smaller portions more often, rather than three full meals a day.

Although giving food may be a way you feel you can nurture your loved one, it's important for you to try not to force him to eat. There are a lot of changes going on in the body, and he needs to decide when he is hungry. Trust that he knows what is best for his body. If you are worried that your loved one isn't eating enough or eating properly, ask the doctor or nurse for an opinion.

This is when it's important for you to encourage her to speak up. Or you can speak up for her. Be honest with the doctor about pain and how it's affecting her routine. It may take more than one talk to feel comfortable about the pain medicines given. Some caregivers worry that they will give their loved one too much medicine. This rarely happens, but it's important for you to talk to the doctor about your fears and concerns.

Talk with the health care team about how to keep your loved one as comfortable as possible. Make sure to include any hospice staff you may have. There are drugs that can help treat pain. These drugs can also be adjusted or changed if they aren't working or have unpleasant side effects.

Don't be afraid to ask for stronger pain relievers or larger doses if the patient needs them. Addiction is not an issue in people with advanced cancer. Instead, they will help your loved one stay as comfortable as possible. People with a history of addiction will want to talk to their doctor about any concerns. For more information, see the NCI booklet, *Pain Control* (see inside cover).

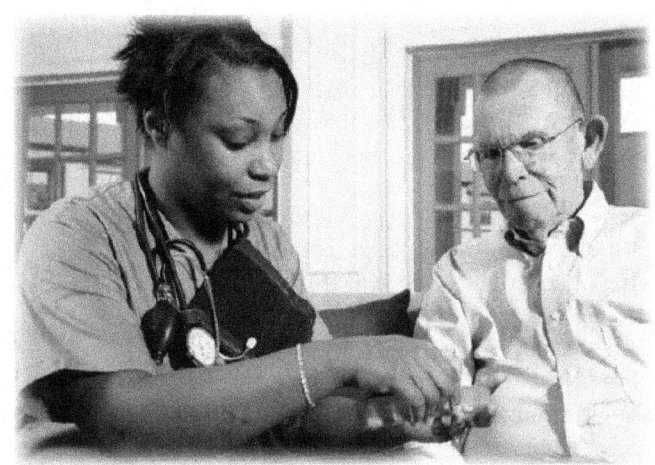

Asking About Other Changes

Sometimes, as treatment continues, changes may take place in the person with cancer. These may be due to the side effects of treatment or the cancer itself. Or they may be caused by other drugs. Some caregivers have said that they wished they had known about these changes sooner. They wished they had known what to expect.

Changes may occur in:

■ Looks

■ Personality or mood

■ Memory

■ Sleep

■ Appetite or nutrition needs

The person you are caring for may or may not go through any of these changes. But you should ask the doctor whether you need to be aware of them. At the same time, ask what you can do about them if they happen. It will help you to know that these changes are normal, and give you ways to be prepared.

Some caregivers who have lost their loved one say they wished they had known the signs that death is near. They say this would have helped them be less afraid or worried. A list of the most common signs is provided on page 52.

"No one told us what steroids would do. My partner started to have mood swings all of a sudden. She'd get really angry at me for no reason. Her nurse told me later this was common when taking these drugs, but how was I supposed to know that?" —Pat

"I remember in the early days my mom had a lot of depression, and I thought it was because of her cancer. But it wasn't—it was the drugs causing it. If I had known about that earlier, I could have dealt with it a lot better." —Debbie

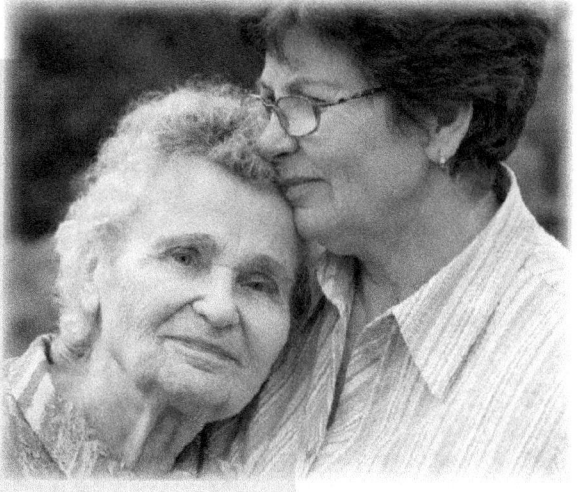

People can refuse treatment at any time. In some states, doctors also have the right to stop aggressive treatment that they don't think is working. If your loved one will be in the hospital, make sure that her wishes for care are clear to you and to the hospital staff. You want the staff to know any measures she wants, or doesn't want, taken if her condition changes. Sometimes this information is not in a patient's chart.

General Tips for Meeting With the Health Care Team

If you are going with the patient to medical visits, here are some general tips for meeting with the health care team:

- Make a list of questions before each appointment.

- Take notes. Or ask the doctor if it's okay to use a tape recorder.

- Get a phone number of someone to call with follow-up questions.

- Keep a file or notebook of all the papers and test results. Make sure it's taken to medical visits.

- Keep records or a diary of all the visits. List the drugs and tests your loved one has taken.

- Keep a record of any upsetting symptoms or side effects. Note when and where they occur.

- Find out what to do in an emergency. This includes who to call, how to reach them, and where to go.

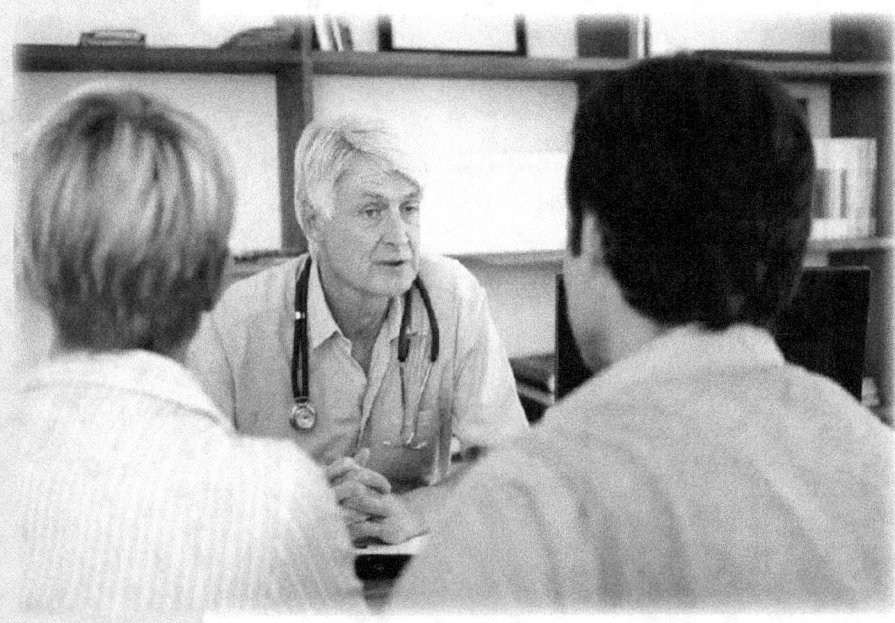

Getting Support

Knowing Your Strengths and Limits

You may be faced with new challenges and concerns now that your loved one has advanced cancer. If the illness has been going on for a long time, these challenges may wear you down even more. Many caregivers say that, looking back, they took on too much themselves. Or they wish they had asked for help sooner in sharing tasks or seeking support. Take an honest look at what you can and can't do. What things are you good at? What do you need to do yourself? What tasks can you give to or share with others? Be willing to let go of things that others can do.

Many people probably want to help but don't know what you need or whether you want help. And as the cancer progresses, you may see changes in the support you get from others. For example:

- People who have helped before may not help now.

- Others who have helped before may want to help in new ways now.

- People who haven't helped before may start helping now.

- Agencies that couldn't help before may offer services now.

> "You have to learn that if people offer, let them do something. Tell them what you need to have done, because they don't know. You have to be willing to let go of your pride and let them help you." —Lynn

Why Getting Help Is Important

Many people don't want support when they need it most, so it's normal to feel this way. You may pull back from your regular social life and people in general. You may feel that it's just too much work to ask for help. Some caregivers have said that more people helped them in the beginning. But as time went on, they felt abandoned.

Accepting help from others isn't always easy. When tough things happen, some people tend to pull away. They think, "We can handle this on our own." But things can get harder as your loved one continues to go through treatment. You may need to change your schedule and take on new tasks. As a result, many caregivers have said, "There's just too much on my plate." They feel stretched to the point that they can't do it anymore. As simple as it sounds, it's good to remind others that you still need help.

> "I have been the main caregiver the whole time. At first, we had emotional support from the church and friends and so on, but over time they have just faded off. I have been stressed beyond belief." —Marion

Keeping a Balance with Visitors

You may have many more people calling you or coming by to visit than ever before. Many caregivers say they feel very blessed when people show they care. Although you probably are very thankful for their love and support, there may be times when you need some space. It's okay if you need time to yourself or just with your family. Some things you can do are:

■ Let your answering machine pick up the messages.

■ Answer the phone in shifts. Take turns with family members or friends to be in charge of calls for a few hours.

■ Put a sign on the door of your home or hospital room thanking people for coming by, but let them know your loved one is resting. Leave room for a note if they want to write one.

■ Have a friend in your home handle visitors while you can be in another part of your home taking care of your own needs.

■ Go to a place where you can't be reached for a while.

Remember that getting help for yourself can also help your loved one, as well as other friends and family.

■ You may stay healthier.

■ Your loved one may feel less guilty about all the things that you're doing.

■ Some of your helpers may offer time and skills that you don't have.

■ Having a support system is a way of taking care of your family. The idea is to remove some tasks so that you can focus on those that you can do.

Talk with someone you trust, such as a friend, member of your faith community, or counselor. Other people may be able to help you sort out your thoughts and feelings. They may also be able to help you find other ways to get support.

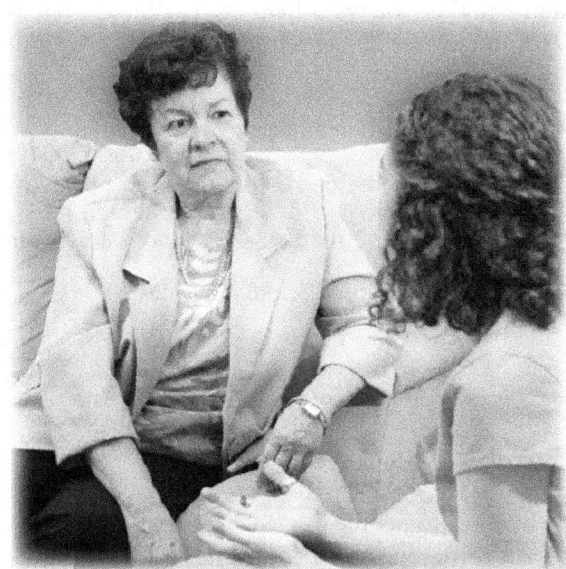

"I was taking on way too much. When I finally asked, more people than I expected were more than willing to help." —Laney

How Can Others Help You?

Many people want to help, but they don't know what you need or how to offer help. It's okay for you to take the first step. Ask for what you need and for the things that would help you most. For instance, you may want someone to:

- Help with household chores, including cooking, cleaning, shopping, yard work, and childcare or eldercare.

- Talk and share your feelings.

- Drive your loved one to appointments.

- Pick up a child from school or activities.

- Pick up a prescription.

- Look up information you need.

- Be the contact person and help keep others updated on your loved one.

> "The people that I had thought would help me weren't there. It was the ones that I really didn't expect to help that were right there saying, 'I'm here for you. What can I do?'" —Antoine

Who Can Help?

Think about people who can help you with tasks. Besides friends and family, think of all the people and groups you and your loved one know. Some examples are neighbors, coworkers, and members of your faith community. The hospital or cancer center may also be able to tell you about services they offer or give you a list of agencies to call. Social workers can also put you in touch with support services.

Be Prepared for Some People to Say "No"

Sometimes, people may not be able to help. This may hurt your feelings or make you angry. It may be especially hard coming from those you expected to help you. You might wonder why someone wouldn't offer to help. Some common reasons are:

- People may be coping with their own problems. Or they may not have enough time.

- People are afraid of cancer or may have already had a bad experience with cancer. They don't want to get involved and feel that pain again.

- Some believe it's best to keep a distance when people are struggling.

- Sometimes people don't realize how hard things really are for you. Or they don't understand that you need help, unless you ask them for it directly.

- Some people feel awkward because they don't know how to show they care.

If people aren't giving you the help you need, you may want to talk to them and explain your needs. Or you can just let it go. But if the relationship is important, you may want to tell the person how you feel. This can help prevent resentment or stress from building up. These feelings could hurt your relationship in the long run.

Long-Distance Caregiving

It can be really tough to be away from your loved one with cancer. You may feel like you're always a step behind in knowing what's happening with care. Yet even if you live far away, it's possible for you to give support and be a care coordinator.

Caregivers who live more than an hour away often rely on the telephone or email as their link. But assessing someone's needs this way can be limiting. You know that you would rush to your loved one's side for a true medical emergency. But other situations are harder to judge. When can you handle things by phone, and when do you need to be there in person?

Finding Contacts

Many caregivers say that it helps to explore both paid and volunteer support. Try to create a support network of people who live near your loved one. These should be people whom you could call day or night and count on in times of crisis. You may also want them to check in with your loved one from time to time.

You could also look into volunteer visitors, adult daycare centers, or meal delivery. Local agencies on aging often list resources online. Checking the white and yellow pages in print or online is useful, too. Give your phone numbers to your loved one's health care team and others for emergencies.

> "My brother is getting worse—he had a bad reaction the other day. I felt so helpless since he was in Colorado and I was here in Georgia. I try to call when I can, but it's so frustrating not knowing for sure what's going on. I don't like feeling so removed."
> —Deondra

Other Tips

- Ask a local family member or friend to update you daily by email. Or, consider creating a website to share news about your loved one's condition and needs.

- Talk to electronic or computer experts about other ways to connect with people. New advances using video and the Internet are being made every day.

- Airlines or bus lines may have special deals for patients or family members. The hospital social worker may also know of other resources, such as private pilots or companies that help people with cancer and their families.

- If you are traveling to see your loved one, time your flights or drives so that you have time to rest when you return. Many long-distance caregivers say that they don't allow themselves enough time to rest after their visits.

- Consider getting a phone card from a discount store to cut down on long-distance bills. Or, review your long-distance and cell phone plans. See if you can make any changes that would reduce your bills.

Life Planning

It's common to feel sad, angry, or worried about lifestyle changes that happen because of your loved one's cancer. You may also be making major decisions that will affect your job or your finances. Finding ways to cope with these issues can bring some peace of mind.

> "I'm not working for the money. I'm working for the benefits. If we don't have benefits, we'd lose everything." —Philip

Handling Money Worries

The financial challenges that people with cancer and their families face are very real. During an illness, you may find it's hard to have enough time or energy to review your options. Yet it's important to keep your family financially healthy.

For hospital bills, you or your loved one may want to talk with a hospital financial counselor. You may be able to work out a monthly payment plan or even get a reduced rate. You should also stay in touch with the insurance company to make sure certain treatment costs are covered.

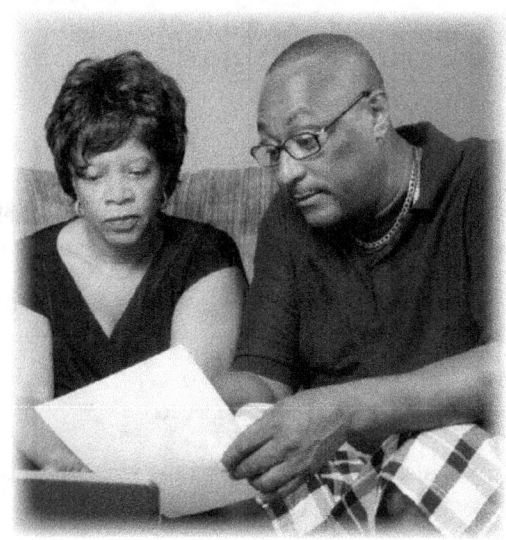

For information about resources that are available, see the Resources section on page 53. You can also get the NCI fact sheet, "Resources for Financial Assistance for Patients and Their Families," at www.cancer.gov, by searching for the terms "financial assistance." Or call toll-free 1-800-4-CANCER (1-800-422-6237) to ask for a free copy.

Coping with Work Issues

One of the greatest sources of strain is trying to balance work demands with providing care and support. The stress of caregiving can have effects on your work life in many ways, such as:

- Causing mood swings that leave coworkers confused or reluctant to work with you

- Making you distracted or less productive

- Causing you to be late or call in sick because of stress

- Creating pressure from being the sole provider for your family if your spouse or partner is unable to work

- Creating pressure to keep working, even though retirement may have been approaching

It's a good idea to check into your company's rules and policies related to a loved one's illness. See if there are any support programs for employees. Many companies have employee assistance programs with work-life counselors for you to talk with. Some companies have eldercare policies or other employee benefit programs that can help support you. Your employer may let you use your paid sick leave or leave without pay.

If your employer doesn't have any policies in place, you could try to arrange something informally. Examples include flex-time, switching shifts with coworkers, adjusting your schedule, or telecommuting as needed.

> "A lot of times I come home from being at the hospital with no sleep and then have to get to work the next morning. It's very tiring." —Betsy

The Family and Medical Leave Act may apply to your situation. Covered employers must give eligible employees up to 12 work weeks of unpaid leave during a 12-month period to care for an immediate family member with a serious health condition. Visit the U.S. Department of Labor website at www.dol.gov/esa/whd/fmla for more information. For sources of support, see the Resources section on page 53.

Looking at Living Arrangements

Sometimes questions are raised about whether a loved one should live alone or with someone else. When making these decisions, here are a few good questions to ask:

- What kind of help does your loved one need?

- Is it risky for her to live alone?

- How often will she need help?

You'll also need to consider how your loved one feels. She may fear:

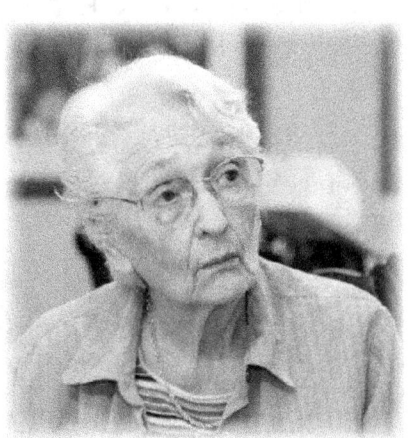

- Losing her independence

- Being seen as weak or a burden to others

- Moving to a health care or other type of assisted living facility

Sometimes it's easier to consider a change in living arrangements when the advice comes from a health professional. Social workers, visiting nurses, those who work with older adults, and others, may be able to help you talk to your loved one.

Advance Directives

If you have not done so already, it's important to start talking with your loved one about his wishes. There may come a time when he can't tell the health care team what he needs. Some people prefer to let their doctor or family members make decisions for them. But often people with cancer feel better once their wishes are known. Talk with your loved one about what kind of care he wants. The more you know, the more prepared you'll be.

Advance directives are legal papers that tell the doctors what to do if your loved one can't tell them himself. The papers let the patient decide ahead of time how he wants to be treated. They may include a living will and a durable power of attorney.

- A **living will** lets people know what kind of medical care patients want if they are unable to speak for themselves.

- A **durable power of attorney for health care** names a person to make medical decisions for a patient when she can't make them herself. This person, chosen by the patient, is called a **health care proxy**. It should be a person she trusts to carry out her decisions and preferences.

Setting up an advance directive is not the same as giving up. Making decisions now keeps the patient in control. This way, his wishes are known and can be followed. This can help everyone worry less about the future and live each day to the fullest.

Make copies of your loved one's advance directives for the health care team and the hospital medical records department. Keep one set for yourself. This will ensure that everyone knows his wishes.

A lawyer is not always needed to fill out these documents. But you may need a notary public. Each state has its own laws concerning living wills and durable powers of attorney. These laws can vary in important details. In some states, a living will or durable power of attorney signed in another state isn't legal. Talk with a lawyer or social worker to get more details. Or look at your state's government website.

You and your loved one may have different opinions about the contents of the advance directives. You should share your opinions, but in the end, it's his choice. If you both can't agree, you may want to ask someone else to guide the conversation between you both. You might talk to a member of your faith community, a social worker, other people dealing with cancer, or a hospice worker.

Other Legal Papers

Here are some other legal papers that are not part of the advance directives:

- A **will** tells how a person wants to divide money and property among heirs (survivors).

- **Legal power of attorney** appoints a person to make financial decisions for the patient when he can't make them.

A Checklist for Organizing Your Loved One's Affairs

- [ ] If your loved one can't physically gather important papers, have her make a list of where you can find them.

- [ ] Keep papers in a fireproof box or with a lawyer.

- [ ] If your loved one keeps important papers in a safe deposit box, he should make sure that a trusted family member or friend has access to it.

- [ ] Although original documents are needed for legal purposes, family members should have photocopies.

- [ ] A worksheet of personal affairs is on page 48. You can use it as a guide to the types of papers your family will need.

Other Planning

Careful planning may reduce the financial, legal, and emotional burden you may face if your loved one dies. For many people, it's hard to bring up these subjects. But talking about them now can help you avoid problems later.

Maybe you don't feel comfortable bringing up the subject. Or maybe your family simply doesn't talk about these things. In either case, seek help from a member of the health care team. They may be able to help your loved one and your family understand the importance of talking about these issues early.

- **Clearing up insurance issues.** Contact the health insurance company if the patient decides to try a new treatment or get hospice care. Most insurance plans cover hospice. They also cover brief home visits from a nurse or home health aide several times a week. But it's wise to ask in advance. This may prevent payment problems later.

- **Putting affairs in order.** You can help your loved one by making sure that he organizes his records, insurance policies, documents, and instructions. He may want to call his bank to make sure that he has taken all the right steps.

- **Talking about funeral wishes.** Some people plan services that are celebrations. Others prefer more traditional services. You and your loved one may want to plan a funeral or memorial service together. It may help both of you to plan a ceremony that meets her desires and has her personal touch.

Talking with Family and Friends

Talking about serious issues is never easy. It's hard to face an uncertain future and the potential death of your loved one. Often people are uncomfortable talking about it, or just don't know what to say. But you will need to talk to your loved one or others about a number of issues. These might include the seriousness of the cancer, preparing for the future, fears of death, or wishes at the end of life.

Some families talk openly about things. Others don't. There is no right or wrong way to communicate. But studies show that families who talk things out feel better about the care they get and the decisions they make.

"My brother doesn't want to make any decisions about his treatment. He has left it up to the rest of us and doesn't want to know anything. So we just sit down with the doctor and go over all the options and try to do the best we can." —Marcus

Talking with Your Loved One Who Has Advanced Cancer

It's likely that you and your loved one are both having the same thoughts and fears about the end of life. It's natural to want to protect each other. But talking about death does not cause someone to die. And keeping things to yourself doesn't make them live longer.

You and your loved one can still have hope for longer life or an unexpected recovery. But it's also a good idea to talk about what's happening and the fact that the future is uncertain. And keeping the truth from each other isn't healthy. Avoiding important issues only makes them harder to deal with later. You may find that you both are thinking the same things. Or you may find you're thinking very different things. This makes it all the more important to get them out in the open. Talking over your concerns can be very healing for all involved.

Often the best way to communicate with someone is to just listen. This is one of the main ways of showing that you're there for them. It may be one of the most valuable things you can do. And it's important to be supportive of whatever your loved one wants to say. It's his life and his cancer. He needs to process his thoughts and fears in his own time and his own way. You can always ask whether he is willing to think about the issue and talk another time. He may even prefer to talk to someone else about the topic.

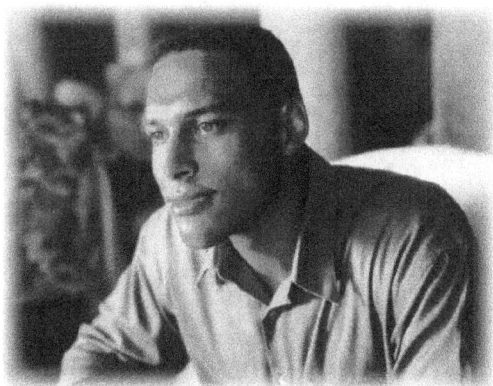

Bringing Up Hard Topics

Bringing up challenging subjects is draining. You may think, for example, that your loved one needs to try a different treatment or see a different doctor. Or she may be worrying about losing independence, being seen as weak, or being a burden to you.

What is important to remember is that your loved one has the right to choose how to live the rest of her life. Although you may have strong opinions about what she should do, the decision is hers to make. Here are some tips on how to bring up hard topics:

- Practice what you'll say in advance.

- Find a quiet time. Ask if it's an okay time to talk.

- Be clear on what your aims are. What do you want as the result?

- Speak from your heart.

- Allow time for your loved one to talk. Listen and try not to interrupt.

- Don't feel the need to settle things after one talk.

- You don't always have to say, "It'll be okay."

Some people won't start a conversation themselves, but may respond if you start first. Also, you can ask other caregivers how they have handled hard topics.

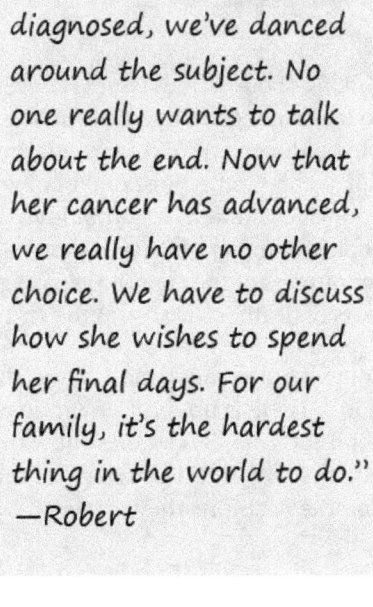

"Ever since Audrey was diagnosed, we've danced around the subject. No one really wants to talk about the end. Now that her cancer has advanced, we really have no other choice. We have to discuss how she wishes to spend her final days. For our family, it's the hardest thing in the world to do."
—Robert

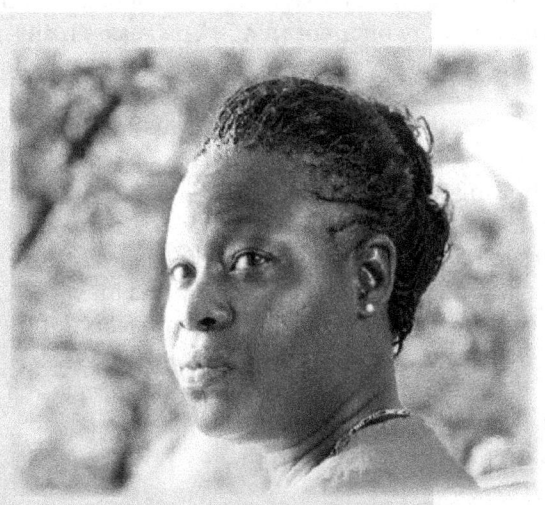

"There was so much we wanted to say to John, but we didn't know how to find the words. So a friend of ours who's a nurse helped us set up an evening with the whole family in John's room, and each of us told him how much we loved him. Having that time together with him meant so much to us." —Kiesha

If you continue to have trouble talking about painful issues, ask for professional advice. A mental health expert may be able to help you explore issues that you don't feel you can yourselves. But if your loved one doesn't want to go, you can always make an appointment to go alone. You may hear some ideas for how to bring up these topics. You can also talk about other concerns and feelings that you are dealing with right now.

Words to Try*	
When You Think You Want to Say...	**Try This Instead:**
Dad, you are going to be just fine.	Dad, are there some things that worry you?
Don't talk like that! You can beat this!	It must be hard to come to terms with all this.
I can't see how anyone can help.	We will be there for you always.
I just can't talk about this.	I am feeling a little overwhelmed right now. Can we take this up later tonight?
What do the doctors know? You might live forever.	Do you think the doctors are right? How does it seem to you?
Please don't give up. I need you here.	I need you here. I will miss you terribly. But we will get through somehow.
There has to be something more to do.	Let's be sure to get the best of medical treatments, but let's be together when we have done all we can.
Don't be glum. You'll get well.	It must be hard. Can I just sit with you for a while?

* From Lynn, J. and J. Harrold. 2011. *Handbook for Mortals: Guidance for People Facing Serious Illness*. Oxford University Press: New York, NY. Reprinted with permission.

Talking with Children and Teens

"This is the only childhood they will ever have, a crucial time of development. Choose to see your illness not as an obstacle but as a powerful platform from which your messages are amplified, helping your children understand and believe you and feel your love in a powerful way... When the facts are couched in love and hopefulness, you can guide your children toward a life-enhancing perception of reality."
—Wendy Harpham, MD*

Children as young as 18 months begin to think about and understand the world around them. If someone close to them has advanced cancer, their world may be changing monthly, weekly, or daily. That's why it's important to be honest with them and prepare them each step of the way. Children need to be reassured that they will be taken care of no matter what happens.

Your own daily stresses and fears can affect how you act with your kids. You may be torn between wanting to give time to your kids, and knowing your loved one with cancer also needs your time. That's why it's good to let children know how you're feeling, as well as to find out how they're feeling. And never assume you know what your children are thinking. You can't predict how they will react to information, either. Experts say that telling children the truth about the cancer is better than leaving their imaginations free to worry about the worst.

Although it's a very hard chapter in a family's life, children can continue to grow and learn during this time. Dealing with cancer honestly and openly can teach them how to handle uncertainty for the rest of their lives. Making the most of the present is an important lesson for everyone to learn.

* Harpham, W. 2004. *When A Parent Has Cancer: A Guide to Caring For Your Children*. New York, NY; Harper Paperbacks. Adapted with permission.

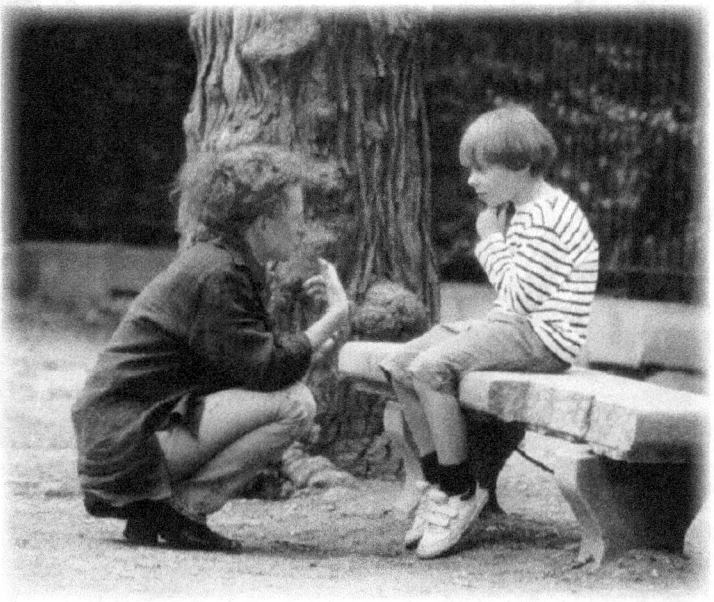

Keeping the Lines of Communication Open

Understand Your Children's Actions and Feelings

Children react to their loved one's cancer in many different ways. They may:

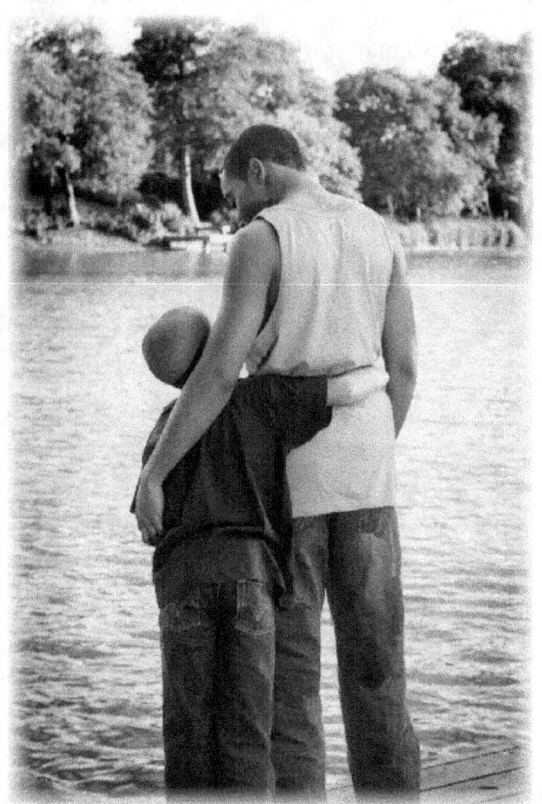

- Seem confused, scared, angry, lonely, or overwhelmed

- Feel scared or unsure how to act when they see the treatment's effects on the patient

- Act clingy or miss all the attention they used to get

- Feel responsible or guilty

- Get angry if they're asked to do more chores around the house

- Get into trouble at school and neglect their homework

- Have trouble eating, sleeping, keeping up with schoolwork, or relating to friends

- Be angry that someone else is taking care of them now

No matter how your children are reacting, it's usually easier to deal with their feelings before problems appear. If they don't open up to you, they may prefer talking to someone outside the family, such as a trusted teacher or coach. If you notice changes or problems, you may want to ask for help from your pediatrician who knows your family already, the school counselor, a social worker or a child life specialist. Any of these may be able to suggest a mental health professional for your children, if needed.

Other Behaviors

It's normal for some children to show signs of regression. They may begin acting younger than their years, resuming behaviors that they had stopped, such as babytalk or bedwetting. Or they may lose skills they had mastered recently. This is usually a sign of stress. Regression indicates that your children need more attention. It's a way for them to express their feelings and, in their own way, ask for support. Recognize that they are needier right now. Be patient as you work with them to get them back to their normal behavior. But don't hesitate to seek help from a social worker or other professional if you need more advice or support.

Try to Ask Open-Ended Questions

For some families, talking about serious issues is very difficult. As challenging as it may be, *not* talking about it can be worse. Try to ask open-ended questions, instead of "yes" or "no" questions. Here are some ideas you might want to share with children of any age:

- "No matter what happens, you will always be taken care of."

- "Nothing you did caused the cancer. And there is nothing you can do to take it away either."

- "People may act differently around you because they're worried about you or worried about all of us."

- "You can ask me anything anytime."

- "Are you okay talking with me about this? Or would you rather talk to Mrs. Jones at school?"

- "It is okay to be upset, angry, scared, or sad about all this. You may feel lots of feelings throughout this time. You'll probably feel happy sometimes, too. It's okay to feel all those things."

Encourage Your Children to Share Their Feelings and Questions

Let children know they're not alone, and it's normal to have mixed emotions. Help them find ways to talk about their feelings. Young children may be able to show you how they're feeling by playing with dolls or drawing pictures. Other forms of art can help older children express themselves. Keep encouraging them to ask questions throughout caregiving. Keep in mind that young children may ask the same question over and over. This is normal, and you should calmly answer the question each time.

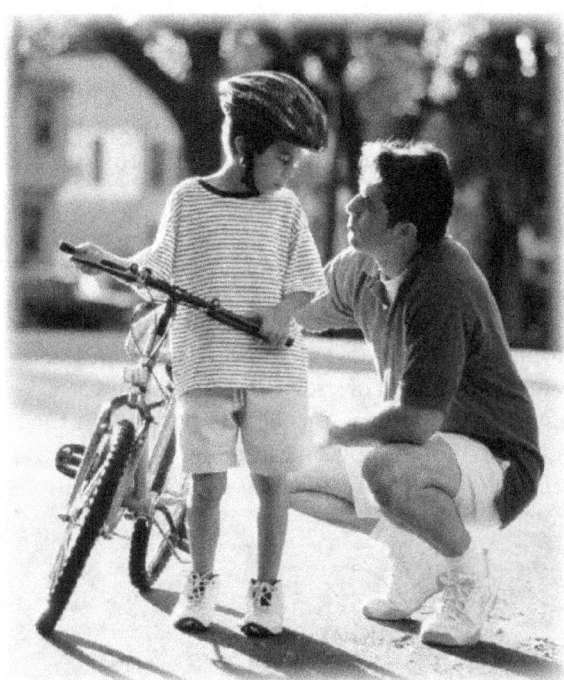

Find Moments to Connect

Come up with new ways to connect. Make a point of tucking them in at bedtime, eating together, reading to them, talking on the phone or by email. Talk to them while you fold clothes or do the dishes. Have a set time when your children do homework while you do something else in the same room. Or take a walk together. Going to the grocery store can even be "together time." Just 5 minutes alone with each child without interruptions can make a world of difference.

Find Others to Help Out

It may be very hard to give your children the time and energy that you normally would. But despite what's going on, they still need to follow a normal routine as much as possible. They need to bathe, eat, play, and spend time with others. Are your children close to another adult, such as a teacher, coach, or some other person? If so, maybe you can ask them to help you with your kids while you handle your extra responsibilities.

You can also call on your own close friends to help out with some tasks, such as cooking dinner or taking the kids out for a pizza. These may be people your kids know well and are comfortable being with. You could ask others who don't know them as well to help with smaller tasks, such as carpooling or bringing meals over.

Talking with Teens

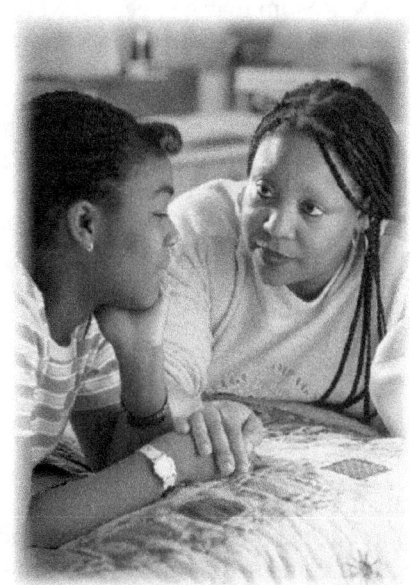

Teens may ask very tough questions, or questions for which you don't have answers. They may ask the "what if" questions and what cancer means for the future. As always, keep being honest with them. Even more important, listen to what they have to say. As with adults, sometimes it's the listening that counts, not the words you speak to them.

Older children, especially teenagers, may feel uncomfortable sharing their feelings with you. They may try to ignore or avoid topics. Encourage them to talk with others. Also let them know that it's okay if they don't know what they're feeling right now. Many older children also find comfort in just spending time together, without talking about the situation. Hugs and letting your children know that you understand can help.

With teenagers, problems may be less obvious or more complicated than with younger children. Here are some things to keep in mind:

- Teens are supposed to be starting to be more independent from their families. Cancer makes this harder to do, leading some teens to act out or withdraw.

- Teens may give off the message of "leave me alone" when they still need and want your attention and support.

- Being a teen under normal circumstances is stressful. Some moods you see may have nothing to do with the family illness.

- Teens want to feel "normal." Make sure they have time for regular activities.

- Keep the communication lines open and involve your teens in decisions as much as possible. Make sure they have a safe place to talk about what is going on in their life. If it's hard for you to be on top of their activities and feelings right now, involve another responsible adult to be closely connected with your teens.

Preparing Children for Visits

If your children don't live with the person who has cancer, it's helpful to prepare them before they visit. The decision of whether or not to let them visit is up to you, your loved one, and perhaps other family members. However, children should have the choice about whether or not they want to go see the patient. If she is in a hospital or other facility, explain what the area and the room look like. Tell them who might be there and what they might see. Also explain gently if her physical condition or personality has changed.

For a younger child, you might say something like this:

- "Grandma is very sick. When you see her, she will be in bed. She may not have a lot of energy to play with you or talk as much. She may look a little different, too."

- "Mom may be sleeping while you're there. Or she may be awake but won't talk because she's resting. But she'll know and be happy that you're there. She loves you!"

- "Don't worry if you're visiting Uncle Bill and he says things that don't make sense. Sometimes the medicine he takes makes him do that. If it happens, we can tell his doctor about it to make sure he's okay."

Sometimes children don't want to visit, or can't for other reasons. In that case, there are other ways of showing they care. They can write a letter or do artwork. They can call the patient up or leave messages or songs on an answering machine. Encourage them to show love and support in any way they want.

Talking to Children About Death

Children deserve to be told the truth about a poor prognosis. Hiding the truth from them leaves them unprepared for the loved one's death and can prolong the grief they will feel. And if you don't talk about the loved one's condition or don't tell the truth about it, you risk your children having difficulty trusting others when they grow up. By including children in the family crisis, you can guide your children toward healthy ways of coping with what is happening and help them prepare for their impending loss in healing ways.

Children of all ages may wonder about dying, life after death, and what happens to the body. It's important to answer all their questions. If not, they may imagine things that are worse than reality. Let them know that everything is being done to keep their loved one comfortable. Tell them that you will keep them updated. And provide opportunities for them to say good-bye.

In order to answer these difficult life questions, you need to know your own views on these subjects. What are you hoping for? What do you think will happen? You can show them how to hope for the best while accepting and preparing for the likely outcome (of death). If you're honest and up front, you are teaching them that death is a natural part of life. It shows them it's okay to talk about it. It can also be a time for them to be reminded that they won't be alone in their time of need. You will always be there for them.

Counselors and oncology social workers can help you handle these questions, too. They may know of local or national programs that offer help to children in these situations. Or they may suggest books, videos, and websites that explore these topics.

Communicating With Your Partner with Cancer

Some couples feel more comfortable talking about serious issues than others. Only you and your partner know how you feel about it.

Some things that cause stress for you and your partner can't be solved right now. But sometimes talking about them can be helpful. You may want to say something like this up front, "I know we can't solve this today. But I'd like to just talk some about how it's going and how we're feeling."

Topics to explore may include how each person:

- Copes with change and the unknown

- Feels about being a caregiver or being cared for

- Handles changing roles in the relationship or home

- Would like to be connected to one another

- Sees what issues may be straining the relationship

- Feels, or would like to feel, cared for and appreciated

- Feels thankful for the other person

> "I've noticed that my husband tries to stay really positive with everyone else, even his parents. He'll say he's doing great. This is frustrating for me because at home, I see that he isn't." —Emily

As your loved one becomes sicker, you may also want to share more practical issues. These may include which decisions you should share together, and which you should make alone. Along with this, you may want to talk about the different tasks you can each handle right now.

Find Ways to Say Thanks

Maybe your partner used to do a lot to keep your family going. And now, because he's sick, you're trying to get used to less help. It may be hard to notice the small things your partner is still doing to help out. There's often too much going on. But when you can, try to look for these things and thank your partner for doing them.

Often it doesn't take much to put a bright spot in your loved one's day. Bringing your partner a cool drink, giving him a card, or calling to check in can show him that you care. Showing a little gratitude can make both of you feel better.

Spend Time Together

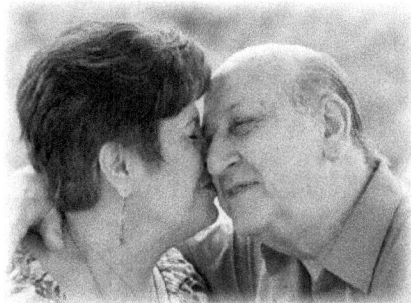

Many couples find that it helps to plan special time together. Some days may be better than others, depending on how your partner feels. So you may need to be okay with last-minute changes. You don't have to be fancy. It's about spending time together. That can mean watching a video, going out to eat, or looking through old photos. It can be whatever you both like to do. You also can plan occasions to include other people, if you miss that.

Communication Troubles

Studies show that open and caring communication works best. Yet often caregivers run into:

- Tension from different ways of communicating

- Lack of sensitivity or understanding about appropriate ways to talk and share feelings

- People who don't know what to say, won't communicate at all, or won't be honest

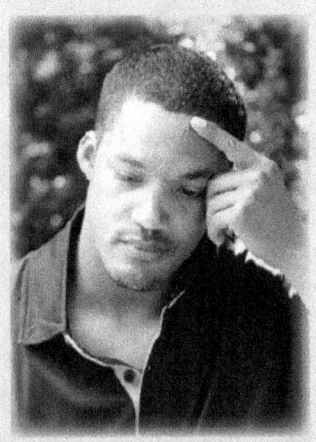

Find Ways to Be Intimate

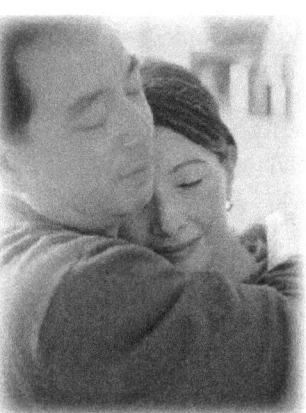

You may find that your sex life with your partner is different than it used to be. Many things could be affecting it:

- Your partner is tired, in pain, or uncomfortable.

- You're tired.

- Your relationship feels distant or strained.

- You or your partner may not be comfortable with the way he or she looks.

- You may be afraid of hurting your partner.

- Your partner's treatment might be affecting his or her interest in sex or ability to perform.

You can still have an intimate relationship in spite of these issues. Intimacy isn't just physical. It also involves feelings. Here are some ways to keep your intimate relationship:

- **Talk about it.** Choose a time when you both can talk. Focus on how you can renew your connection.

- **Try not to judge.** If your partner isn't performing, try not to read meaning into it. Let your partner tell you what he or she needs.

- **Make space.** Protect your time together. Turn off the phone and TV. If needed, find someone to take care of the kids for a few hours.

- **Reconnect.** Plan an hour or so to be together without trying to have sex. For example, you may want to play special music or take a walk. Take it slow. This time is about reconnecting.

- **Try new touch.** Cancer treatment or surgery can change your partner's body. Areas where touch used to feel good may now be numb or painful. For now, you can figure out together what kind of touch feels good, such as holding, hugging, and cuddling.

Communicating with Other Family Members and Friends

Any problems your family may have had before the cancer diagnosis are likely to be more intense now. This is true whether you are caring for a young child, an adult child, a parent, or a spouse. Your caregiver role can often trigger feelings and role changes that affect your family in ways you never expected. And relatives you don't know very well or who live far away may be present more often, which may complicate things.

It's very common for families to argue over a number of things at this time. These might include:

- Treatment options for their loved one, or whether to continue treatment at all

- When to use hospice care

- What treatment the patient desires

- Feelings that some family members help more than others

While everyone may be trying to do what's best for your loved one, some family members may disagree as to what this means. Everyone brings their own set of beliefs and values to the table, which makes these decisions hard. It is often during these times that families ask their health care team to hold a family meeting.

Family Meetings

Family meetings are necessary throughout cancer care. They become even more important as cancer progresses. In a family meeting, the health care team and family meet to discuss care. You can ask a social worker or counselor to be there if needed. Talk with your loved one to see if he wants a family meeting. Ask if he would like to be involved. Meetings can be used to:

> "My sisters keep hoping for the magic bullet. I don't know how to get them to understand how serious things are." —Verdell

- Have the health care team explain the overall goals for care

- Let the family state their wishes for care

- Give everyone an open forum in which to express their feelings

- Clarify caregiving tasks

If you need to, bring a list of issues to discuss. At the end of the meeting, ask the health care team to summarize decisions and plan next steps.

How to Communicate When Support Isn't Useful

Sometimes people are eager to help you because they want to feel useful. But at times you may not need the support, or you may simply want to spend time alone with your sick loved one.

If people offer help that you don't need or want, thank them for their concern. Let them know that right now you have things under control, but you'll contact them if you need anything. You can tell them that it always helps to send cards, letters, and emails. Or they can pray or send good thoughts.

Sometimes people offer unwanted advice on parenting, medical care, or any number of issues. It can be unpleasant to hear such comments. For example, some caregivers have shared:

- "We have a problem with a member of my husband's family. She doesn't live here and keeps questioning all our decisions. It's gotten so bad that we've had our doctor explain to her that she's not here all day, and, therefore, doesn't understand the situation. She has been a real pain."

- "I feel like people really want him to do the treatment they are suggesting, rather than what we feel is best. It's making this harder than it needs to be."

People often offer unwanted advice because they aren't sure what else they can do. They may feel helpless to do anything, yet want to show their concern. While it may come from a good place, it can still seem judgmental to you.

It's your decision on how to deal with these opinions. You don't have to respond at all if you don't want to. If someone has concerns about your kids that seem valid, talk to a counselor or teacher about what steps to take. Or if the concerns are about your loved one, you can talk to the medical team. Otherwise, thank them. And reassure them that you are taking the necessary steps to get your loved one and family through this tough time.

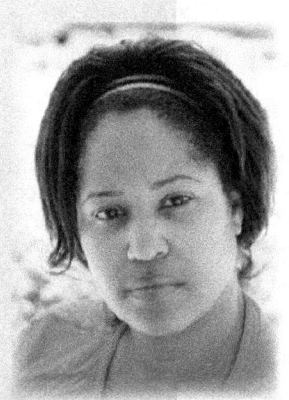

"My mother came by and commented on how much television the kids were watching. She made some remark about how she knew I was stressed, but couldn't I find something better for them to do? I told her I've got a lot on my mind, and needed her understanding right now." —Carrie

Coping with Your Feelings

You've probably had a range of feelings as you care for your loved one. These emotions can be quite strong at times and less so at others. It takes a lot of energy to stay hopeful and cope with the ongoing waves of emotion. Now that the cancer has advanced, these feelings may be even more intense.

Guilt

Feeling guilty is a common reaction for caregivers. You may worry that you aren't helping enough, or that your work or distance from your loved one is getting in the way. You may even feel guilty that you are healthy. Or you may feel guilty for not acting upbeat or cheerful. But know that it's okay. You have reasons to feel upset, and hiding them may keep other people from understanding your needs.

> "Some days I'm stressed beyond belief. Then other days I feel thankful for the time I have spent with my wife all these years. Then the next day, I feel angry that I have to juggle so much, and then I feel guilty for being angry. Basically, I never know how I'm going to feel one day to the next." —Jim

Hope or Hopelessness

You may feel hope or hopelessness to different degrees throughout the cancer treatment. Your hopes and dreams change with time, and shift back and forth. Although remission may no longer be possible for your loved one, it's okay to hope for other things. You can hope that you and your loved one experience comfort, peace, acceptance, and even joy in the days ahead. As a caregiver, these feelings of hope may help you get through the next 5 minutes or the next 5 days.

Sadness or Worry

You may feel sad or worried as you watch your loved one struggle with cancer. You may be concerned with how he is coping with side effects or coping with fear. Or you may be worried about bills, your family, or ending up alone.

It's okay to cry or express your feelings when you are alone or with a trusted friend. You don't have to be upbeat all the time or pretend to be cheerful. Give yourself time to cope with the changes you and your loved one may be going through.

> "There are times when you don't know how to help. You can't take away the pain. You can't take away the frustration. All you can do is be there, and it's a very helpless feeling." —Cecile

Anxiety or Depression

Anxiety means you have extra worry, you can't relax, you feel tense, or you have panic attacks. Many people worry about how to pay bills, how things will affect the family, and, of course, how their loved one is coping. Depression is a persistent sadness that lasts more than two weeks. If any of these symptoms start affecting your ability to function normally, talk with your health care provider. Don't think that you need to tough it out without any help. It's likely that your symptoms can be eased. See page 45 for some warning signs of depression.

Grief

Grief is the process of letting go and accepting and learning to live with loss. Part of the grieving process is feeling extreme sadness, as well as other feelings. You may feel sad about the losses you've experienced, including the loss of the life you used to have.

> "I think there's a great deal of preparation being done now, almost advanced bereavement. Sometimes I feel myself grieving her and she's not even gone yet."
> —Artie

But grieving doesn't mean that you have to feel a certain way. Everyone is different. Let yourself grieve in your own way and time. For example, some people may not show as much emotion as others do when they grieve. They show their feelings by doing things, rather than talking about them. This doesn't mean that they aren't feeling "the right way" or that they need to change how they react.

You may begin to feel the loss of your loved one even before he dies. This is called **anticipatory grief**. It's normal to feel sad about the changes you are going through and the losses you are going to have. You may have expected your life with your friend or family member to be different than what you are going through. Feeling sad over what might have been or what is to come is expected. It's normal for you to have grief over the future loss of your loved one and all the changes involved.

Understand that these feelings are normal. And grief can come up at times when you're not expecting it. Although it can come and go in intensity, grief can last for many months. It's important to seek help from hospice staff, a mental health expert, or a support group.

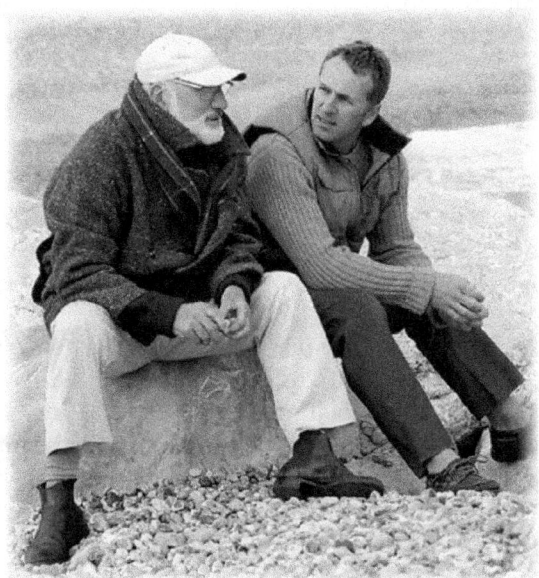

Hurt Feelings

You may be feeling more sensitive right now. Being tired and stressed can put you on edge more than usual. And because of this, your feelings may get hurt more easily. This could be because you feel like you're not being helped enough. Or it could be that you feel people don't understand how much you're going through. However, one common cause of hurt feelings is when the person you're caring for directs anger at you. She may feel stressed, tired, or scared, and in turn, take her anger out on you. Or sometimes medicine causes people to have more anger than they normally would. Try not to take this personally. Ask the doctor if anger is a side effect of medicine. You may also find it helpful to share your feelings with your loved one. Sometimes patients don't realize the effect that their anger has on others. But most of all, remember that we often show our feelings, good or bad, to the people we love the most.

> "It's emotionally exhausting, and I never know what to expect. One minute, things are looking up, and a couple of hours later, something happens and I don't have the answers." —Beth

Anger

Many things are going on right now that can make you angry. You may be angry with yourself, your family, God, or even the person you're caring for. At first, anger can help by moving you to take action. You may decide to learn more about different treatment options or get more medical opinions. But anger doesn't help if you hold it in too long or take it out on others.

It may help to pinpoint why you are angry. This isn't always easy. Sometimes anger comes from feelings that are hard to show, such as fear, panic, or worry. Or it may come from resentment. If these feelings remain, seek help from a counselor or other mental health professional.

Loneliness

You can still feel alone in your role as a caregiver, even if you have lots of people around you. It's easy to feel like no one understands what you're going through. You also may feel lonely because you have less time to see people and do the things you're used to doing. Whatever your situation, you aren't alone. Other caregivers know how you feel and share your feelings. See the Resources section on page 53 for resources you can use to connect with others.

Denial

You may have trouble accepting that your friend or family member may not recover. You may think that if she keeps getting treatment, something may finally work, or a new discovery will be made. There's nothing wrong with this. But try to listen to your loved one and the doctor to really hear what they're saying. Your way of coping may make the patient feel that you don't really understand what's happening. Again, it's okay to deal with things at your own pace. But be aware of the effect this may have on others.

Caring for Your Mind and Spirit

Find Comfort

Your mind needs a break from the demands of caregiving. Think about what gives you comfort or helps you relax. Caregivers say that even a few minutes a day without interruptions helps them to cope and focus.

Take 15–30 minutes each day to do something for yourself, no matter how small it is. (See "Small Things I Can Do for Me" on page 39.) For example, caregivers often find that they feel less tired and stressed after light exercise. Try to make time for taking a walk, going for a run, riding a bike, or doing gentle stretches.

You may find that it's hard to relax even when you have time for it. Some caregivers find it helpful to do exercises designed to help you relax, such as stretching or yoga. Other relaxing activities include taking deep breaths or just sitting still.

Look for Positives

It can be hard finding positive moments when you're busy caregiving. Caregivers say that looking for the good things in life helps them feel better. Each day, try to think about something that you find rewarding about caregiving. You also might take a moment to feel good about anything else from the day that is positive—a nice sunset, a hug, or something funny that you heard or read.

Find Acceptance

You're on your own path toward accepting the fact that your loved one may die. Although it may take time, acceptance can bring feelings of peace. You may find that cancer helps you value life more. You may feel that you live each day more fully, even though the future is unknown.

> "I have gotten a lot of patience from caregiving. I learned it's okay for me to have all the feelings I'm having and for her to have all the ones she's having. I see that we both go through a lot."
> —Esther

Feel Thankful

You may feel thankful that you can be there for your loved one. You may be glad for a chance to do something positive and give to another person in a way you never knew you could. Some caregivers feel that they've been given the chance to build or strengthen a relationship. This doesn't mean that caregiving is easy or stress-free. But finding meaning in caregiving can make it easier to manage.

Connect with Other People

Studies show that connecting with other people is very important for most caregivers. It's especially helpful when you feel overwhelmed. Sometimes you want to say things that you just can't say to your loved one.

Try to find someone you can really open up to about your feelings or fears. You may find it helpful to talk with someone outside the situation. Some caregivers have an informal network of people to contact. Some also see a counselor or a therapist. If you're concerned about a caregiving issue, you may want to talk with your loved one's health care team. Knowledge often helps reduce fears.

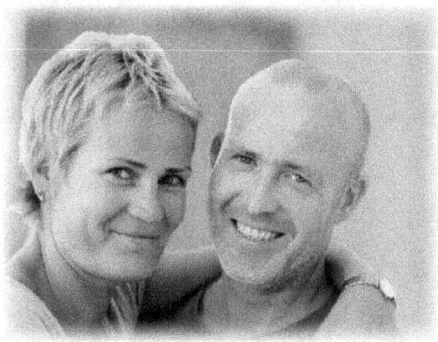

Let Yourself Laugh

It's okay to laugh, even if your loved one has advanced cancer. In fact, it's healthy. Laughter releases tension and makes you feel better. You can read funny columns and comics, watch comedy shows, or talk with upbeat friends. Or remember funny things that have happened to you in the past. Keeping your sense of humor is a good coping skill.

Write in a Journal

Research shows that writing in a journal can relieve negative thoughts and feelings. It can also help improve your health. You can write about any topic. You might write about your most stressful experiences. Or you may want to express your deepest thoughts and feelings. You can also write about things that make you feel good, or what went well that day. Another technique people use is to write down whatever comes to mind. It doesn't have to make sense or have correct grammar. It just gets all the "jumble" out of your mind and onto the paper.

Confront Your Anger or Frustration

You may find that you're getting more and more angry and frustrated as the person you're caring for gets sicker. It may help to try to process these feelings as they happen, rather than hold them in. Ask yourself what's really causing the anger. Are you tired? Frustrated with medical care? Does your loved one seem demanding? If you can, try to let some time pass before bringing up your feelings. It may also help you to express your anger through exercise, art, or even hitting the bed with a pillow.

"It's okay for a neighbor to ask how I'm doing when they want the answer to be, 'I'm fine.' But when I'm really not fine, all I need is to talk to someone who can understand, or just hear me out. You don't have to have an answer, just listen to me." —Kathy

Let Go of Your Guilt

If you are feeling guilty, here are some things you can do:

- Let go of mistakes. You can't be perfect. No one is. The best we can do is learn from our mistakes and move on. Continue to do the best you can. And try not to expect too much from yourself.

- Put your energy into the things that matter to you. Focus on the things you feel are worth your time and energy. Let the other things go for now. For example, don't fold the clothes when you're tired. Go ahead and rest instead.

- Forgive yourself and others. Chances are good that people are doing what they can. That includes you. Each new moment and new day gives you a chance to try again.

"I get tired and angry because I run myself ragged all day. Then I feel guilty for feeling this way because I'm not the one who is sick. Some days, though, I just can't help it. This can seem like a thankless job that I didn't sign up for." —Hao

Join a Support Group

Support groups can meet in person, by phone, or over the Internet. They may help you gain new insight into what's happening, give you ideas about how to cope, and help you know that you're not alone.

In a support group, people may talk about their feelings and what they have gone through. They may trade advice with each other and help others who are dealing with the same kinds of issues. Some people like to go and just listen. And others prefer not to join support groups at all. Some people aren't comfortable with this kind of sharing.

"What I need at least once or twice a week is to talk to someone or a group of people that are in the same shoes as I am." —Vince

If you feel like you would benefit from outside support such as this but can't get to a group in your area, try a support group on the Internet. Some caregivers say websites with support groups have helped them a lot.

Use Respite Help

Many caregivers say that they wish they had gotten respite help sooner. Some say that they waited out of pride or guilt. Others just didn't think of it earlier.

Respite providers spend time with the patient so you can rest, see friends, run errands, or do whatever you'd like to do. Respite services can also help with the physical demands of caregiving, like lifting your loved one into bed or a chair. If this service sounds useful, you may want to:

- Talk with your loved one about having someone come into your home to help out from time to time. If she seems to resist this request, you may want to ask a friend or family member to help explain why this could be good for both of you.

- Get referrals from friends or health care professionals. Your local agency on aging should also have suggestions.

- Ask the respite helpers what types of tasks they do.

You can get respite help from family, friends, neighbors, coworkers, members of your faith community, government agencies, or nonprofit groups. Whatever you do, remember that you haven't failed as a caregiver if you need help and relief.

"Since we're taking care of Dad at home now, Mom and I take turns running each morning while the other person stays with him. It's the only way I can keep my stress level down through all this."
—Meredith

Small Things I Can Do For Me

Each day, take a short vacation from caregiving:

- Nap

- Exercise

- Keep up with a hobby

- Take a drive

- See a movie

- Work in the yard

- Go shopping

- Catch up on phone calls, letters, or email

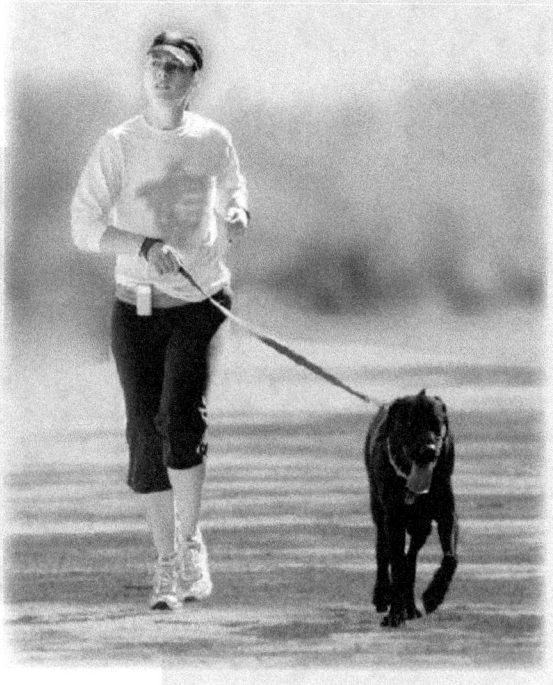

Making Time for Yourself

You may feel that your needs aren't important right now. Or maybe by the time you've taken care of everything else, you have no time left for yourself. Or you may feel guilty that you can enjoy things that your loved one can't right now.

Most caregivers say they have those same feelings. But caring for your own needs, hopes, and desires is important to give you the strength to carry on. (See the "Caregiver's Bill of Rights" on page 47.)

Taking time to recharge your own body, mind, and spirit can help you be a better caregiver. And if you're sick or not feeling well, it's even more important that you take care of yourself, too. You may want to think about:

■ Finding nice things you can do for yourself—even for a few minutes

■ Finding nice things others can do or set up for you

■ Finding new ways to connect with friends

■ Taking larger chunks of time that are "off-duty"

"I just need some quiet time. If my husband's taking a nap, I will read a book or sit on the porch because sometimes it's so intense. We have days where we go straight from chemo to radiation. It's very tiring."
—Adele

Giving yourself an outlet to cope with your thoughts and feelings is important, too. Try to think about what would help give you a lift. Would talking with others help ease your load? Or is quiet time by yourself what you would like best? You might want some of both, depending on what's going on in your life. It's helpful to take the time to think about your own needs.

Finding Meaning

Many caregivers find that the cancer experience causes them to look for meaning in their lives. Taking time to think about your life and your relationship with your loved one may help you feel a sense of closure, accomplishment, and meaning. You may want to share your thoughts with your loved one or others, or you may just want to write them down or tape-record them for yourself.

Here are some questions to ask yourself or your loved one:

- What are the happiest and saddest times we have shared together?

- What are the defining or most important moments of our life together?

- What have we taught each other?

- How has being a caregiver affected my life?

"Before her cancer, I wasn't living my life the way I should have. But when I got the opportunity to take care of my wife, I became really close to her. I've learned things about her I never knew. And we've become really close. I think about life differently, you know. I take it more seriously."
—Armando

When you're ready, you may want to step back and take a further look at life together. When someone you love has cancer, you may begin to rethink the things that are important to you. Some caregivers and their loved ones do things together that they had always planned to do. Others don't make a lot of changes. Instead, they enjoy the life they have together much more. Life can become more about the person, not the disease.

"I have found the cancer gives us a lot of time to spend together. So I ask him questions to find things out about him I didn't know. I wrote a long list out, and each day I ask him a few questions from the list. This has been really special for me and my father. And for my family, too." —Ben

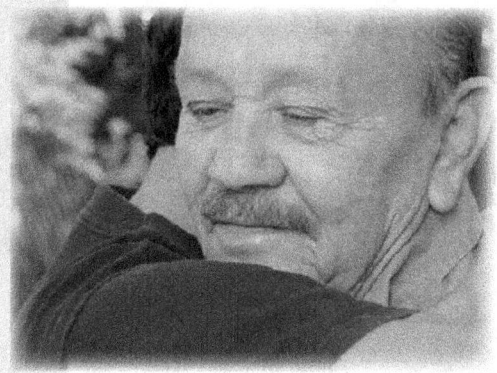

Exploring Spirituality

Questions about the meaning of life and death may come up frequently now. On your own or with your loved one or a close friend, you might consider:

- Why are we here?

- What is a good life to me?

- What is the meaning of my being a caregiver?

- What do I look back on as most positive and negative about my life?

- How has my faith or spirituality helped guide me as a caregiver and as a person?

- How has my faith or spirituality changed during my life?

- Do I have anger or other strong emotions that are directed toward God?

- What kinds of questions do I have that can't be answered?

- Who or what can support me spiritually during this time?

Some things you and your loved one can do to celebrate your life together are:

- Make a video of special memories.

- Review or arrange family photo albums.

- Chart or write down your family's history or family tree.

- Keep a daily journal of feelings and experiences.

- Make a scrapbook.

- Help write notes or letters to other friends and family members.

- Read or write poetry.

- Create artwork, knit, or make jewelry.

- Choose meaningful objects or mementos together to give to others.

- Write down or record funny or meaningful stories from the past.

You, the patient, and other family members can do whatever brings joy and meaning to your lives. Your loved one may even decide to make what is called an "ethical will." It's not a legal paper. It's something a person writes to share with people he or she cares about. Many ethical wills contain the person's thoughts on their values, memories, and hopes. They may also contain the lessons learned in life or other things that are meaningful.

Faith and Spirituality

For some, meaning can be found in religion. Others look to another kind of higher power. Some caregivers wonder why they have to go through this experience. Others feel that they've been blessed by it. Some caregivers feel both these things.

Being spiritual is very personal and means something different for everyone. As you look at life in new ways, you may find a spiritual path helpful. Some ways to add spirituality to your daily life include:

- Reading religious or spiritual books, listening to spiritual music, or watching related videos or TV programs

- Keeping uplifting quotes handy

- Praying or meditating

- Talking with a member of your faith community or someone else with a spiritual nature

- Visiting a place of worship

- Finding a special place where you find beauty or a sense of calm

- Asking the hospital social worker or recreation therapist to suggest relaxing music

> *"I have the utmost respect for people who've been through this or are going through it. It takes a special person to care for somebody. And you know, it really does change your life for the better."* —Louise

Caring for Your Body

You may find yourself so busy and concerned about your loved one that you don't pay attention to your own health. But it's very important that you take care of yourself. Taking care of yourself will give you strength to help others.

Added stress and daily demands often add to any health problems caregivers already have.

They also may have one or more of the problems below:

- Fatigue (tiredness)

- Sleeping problems

- Weaker immune system (poor ability to fight off illness)

- Slower healing of wounds

- Higher blood pressure

- Changes in appetite and/or weight

- Headaches

- Anxiety, depression, or other mood changes

Taking Care of Yourself

These ideas for taking care of yourself may sound easy. But they're a challenge for most caregivers. You'll need to pay attention to how you're feeling, in both body and mind. Even though you're putting your loved one's needs first, it's important to:

- Keep up with your own checkups, screenings, and other medical needs.

- Try to remember to take your medicines as prescribed. Ask your doctor to give you extra refills to save trips. Find out if your grocery store or pharmacy delivers.

- Try to eat healthy meals. Eating well will help you keep up your strength. If your loved one is in the hospital or has long doctor's appointments, bring easy-to-prepare food from home. For example, sandwiches, salads, or packaged foods and canned meats fit easily into a lunch container.

- Get enough rest. Listening to soft music or doing breathing exercises may help you fall asleep. Short naps can energize you if you aren't getting enough sleep. But talk with your doctor if lack of sleep becomes an ongoing problem.

- Exercise. Walking, swimming, running, or bike riding are only a few ways to get your body moving. Any kind of exercise (including working in the garden, cleaning, mowing, or going up stairs) can help you keep your body healthy. Finding at least 15-30 minutes a day to exercise may make you feel better and help manage your stress.

- Make time for yourself to relax. You may choose to stretch, read, watch television, or talk on the phone. Whatever helps you unwind, you should take the time to do it.

Self-Care*

Myths	Facts
"Self-care means that I have to be away from my loved one."	You can do things to take care of yourself with or without your friend or family member in the room with you.
"Taking care of myself takes a lot of time away from other things."	Some self-care only has to take a few minutes, such as reading an upbeat passage or stretching. Other self-care can be done between tasks in free moments.
"I'd have to learn how to do this 'self-care' stuff."	Whatever things make you feel happier, lighter, more relaxed, or more energized count as self-care. Think of things that you already know work for you.

* The Hospice of the Florida Suncoast. "Caring For Yourself While Caring For Others," Adapted with permission.

Do You Need Help with Depression or Anxiety?

Remember, many of the things listed below are normal. This is especially true when you are dealing with a lot of stress. But talk with your doctor if you have any of these signs for more than 2 weeks. Your doctor may have suggestions for treatment.

Changes in Your Feelings

- A feeling of being worried, anxious, "blue," or depressed that does not go away

- Feeling guilty or worthless

- Feeling overwhelmed, out of control, or shaky

- Feeling helpless or hopeless

- Feeling grouchy or moody

- Crying a lot

- Focusing on worries or problems

- Thinking about hurting or killing yourself

- Not being able to get a thought out of your mind

- Not being able to enjoy things (such as food, being with friends, sex)

- Avoiding situations or things that you know are really harmless

- Having trouble concentrating or feeling scatterbrained

- Feeling that you are "losing it"

Body Changes

- Gaining or losing weight without meaning to

- Trouble sleeping or needing more sleep

- Racing heartbeat

- Dry mouth

- Sweating a lot

- Upset stomach

- Diarrhea (loose, watery stools)

- Slowing down physically

- Fatigue (tiredness) that won't go away

- Headache or other aches and pains

Reflection

As a caregiver, you try to strike a balance each day. You have to care for your loved one while keeping up with the demands of family and work. Your focus tends to be on the patient's needs. But it's also up to you to try to stay in tune with yourself. Remember the things you need to maintain a healthy mind, body, and spirit. And if you can, try to find a quiet time for reflection each day. Meditating, praying, or just resting may help you keep a sense of peace at this time.

Caring for someone with advanced cancer has been described by others as the toughest thing they have ever been through. And yet they wouldn't have given it up for the world.

Whether good or bad, life-changing situations often give people the chance to grow, learn, and appreciate what's important to them. Many people who care for someone with cancer describe the experience as a personal journey. They say it has changed them forever. Much like the way people with cancer describe their experience. It's not necessarily a journey that caregivers would have chosen for themselves. But they can use their skills, strength, and talents to support their loved one while finding out more about themselves along the way.

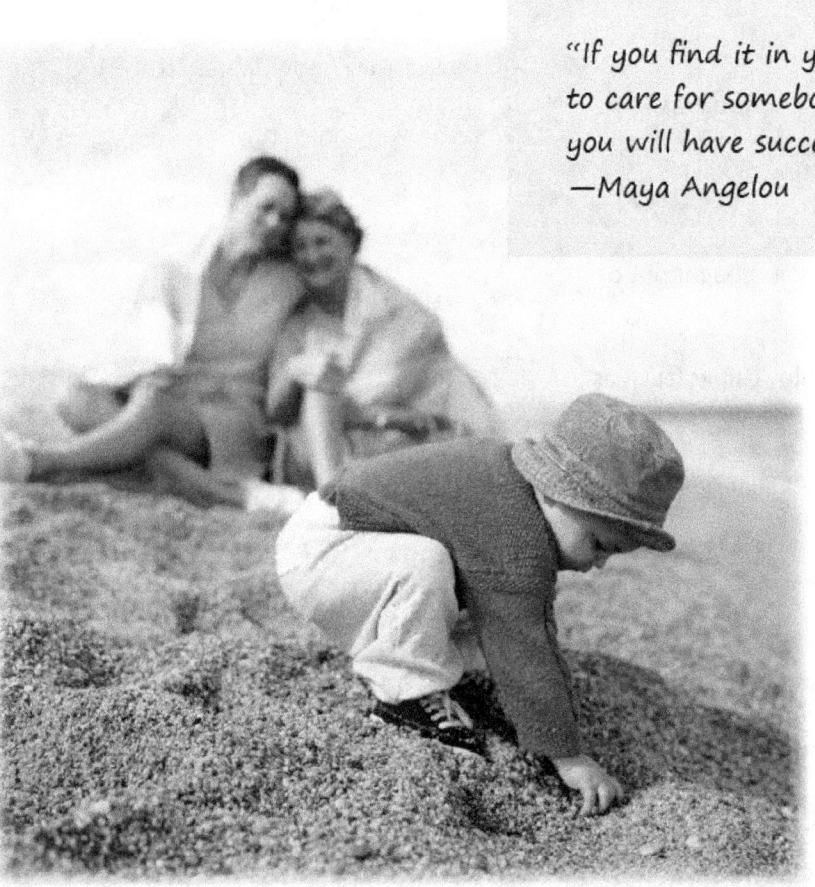

"If you find it in your heart to care for somebody else, you will have succeeded."
—Maya Angelou

Caregiver's Bill of Rights

I have the right to take care of myself. This is not an act of selfishness. It will give me the ability to take better care of my loved one.

I have the right to seek help from others even though my loved one may object. I know the limits of my own endurance and strength.

I have the right to maintain parts of my own life that do not include the person I care for, just as I would if he were healthy. I know that I do everything that I reasonably can do for this person. I have the right to do some things just for myself.

I have the right to get angry, be depressed, and express difficult feelings once in a while.

I have the right to reject any attempt by my loved one to make me do things out of guilt or anger. (It doesn't matter if she knows that she is doing it or not.)

I have the right to get consideration, affection, forgiveness, and acceptance for what I do for my loved one, as I offer these in return.

I have the right to take pride in what I'm doing. And I have the right to applaud the courage it has taken to meet the needs of my loved one.

I have the right to protect my individuality. I also have the right to a life that will sustain me in times when my loved one no longer needs my full-time help.

(Author Unknown)

Personal Affairs Worksheet

You can help your friend or family member with cancer fill out this worksheet. This information may help you manage your loved one's personal affairs. Be sure to let other family members know about this list. It may help all of you cope with your loved one's death and find comfort. It may also be a source of comfort for your loved one, to know that his needs and wishes will be met. Try to keep it updated and in a safe place. Make sure that only those you trust have access to it.

Banks, savings and loans

Contact Information _____

_____

What Needs to be Done _____

_____

Life insurance company

Contact Information _____

_____

What Needs to be Done _____

_____

Health insurance company

Contact Information _____

_____

What Needs to be Done _____

_____

Disability insurance company

Contact Information _____

_____

What Needs to be Done _____

_____

Homeowners' or renters' insurance company

Contact Information _____

_____

What Needs to be Done _____

_____

Burial insurance company

Contact Information _____

_____

What Needs to be Done _____

_____

Unions and fraternal organizations

Contact Information _____

_____

What Needs to be Done _____

_____

Attorney

Contact Information _____

_____

What Needs to be Done _____

_____

Accountant

Contact Information _____

_____

What Needs to be Done _____

_____

Executor of the estate

Contact Information _____

_____

What Needs to be Done _____

_____

Internal Revenue Service

Contact Information _____

_____

What Needs to be Done _____

_____

Social Security office

Contact Information_____

_____

What Needs to be Done _____

_____

Pension or retirement plans

_____

Contact Information_____

_____

What Needs to be Done _____

Department of Veterans Affairs

Contact Information_____

_____

What Needs to be Done _____

_____

Investment companies

Contact Information_____

_____

What Needs to be Done _____

_____

Mortgage companies

Contact Information_____

_____

What Needs to be Done _____

_____

Credit card companies

Contact Information_____

_____

What Needs to be Done _____

_____

All other lenders

Contact Information _____

_____

What Needs to be Done _____

_____

Employer

Contact Information _____

_____

What Needs to be Done _____

_____

Faith or spiritual leader

Contact Information _____

_____

What Needs to be Done _____

_____

Safety deposit box keys and box location

_____

_____

_____

_____

Safe locations and lock combinations

_____

_____

_____

_____

Location of other important items (such as jewelry)

_____

_____

_____

_____

Signs That Death Is Near and What You Can Do

Certain signs and symptoms can help a caregiver know when death is near. They are described below, along with suggestions on how to manage them. It's important to know that not every patient has all of these signs or symptoms. Also, even if any of them are present, it doesn't always mean that your loved one is close to death. A member of the patient's health care team can give you more guidance about what to expect.

Drowsiness, sleeping more, or being unresponsive: Plan visits for times when your loved one is alert. It's important to speak directly to the patient and talk as if he can hear, even if there is no response. Most patients are still able to hear after they're no longer able to speak. Don't try to arouse or shake the patient if he doesn't respond.

Confusion about time, place, and/or identity of friends and family members: Your loved one may also seem restless, or have visions of people and places that are not present. Or she may see, hear, and talk to loved ones who have died. She also may pull at bed linens or clothing. Gently remind her of the time, date, and people who are present. Try to be calm and reassuring. These should not be treated as hallucinations. You don't need to convince her that her visions aren't real.

Being more withdrawn and less social: Speak to your loved one directly. Let him know you are there for him. He may be aware and able to hear, but unable to respond. Some experts say that giving the patient permission to "let go" can be helpful.

Less need for food and liquids, and loss of appetite: Allow your loved one to choose if and when to eat or drink. Ice chips, water, or juice may be refreshing if she can swallow. Lip balm may help to keep the mouth and lips moist.

Loss of bladder or bowel control: Keep your loved one clean, dry, and as comfortable as possible. Place disposable pads on the bed beneath the patient, so you can remove them when they become soiled.

Dark urine or decreased amount of urine: You can ask a doctor or nurse about the need for a catheter. A member of the health care team can teach you how to take care of it if one is needed.

Skin becomes cool to the touch or bluish in color: It's okay to use blankets to warm your loved one. Avoid warming with electric blankets or heating pads, which can cause burns. Take comfort knowing that even though the skin may be cool, the patient is probably not aware of feeling cold.

Rattling or gurgling sounds while breathing: These may seem loud or may seem irregular and shallow. Your loved one may also breathe fast and then slow. Turning his body to the side and placing pillows under the head and behind the back may help. Although this kind of breathing may seem scary to you, it doesn't cause discomfort to your loved one. An extra source of oxygen may help. If he can swallow, ice chips also may help. A cool mist humidifier may help as well.

Turning the head toward a light source: Leaving soft, indirect lights on in the room may help.

Becoming harder to control pain: It's important to keep providing the pain medicines your loved one's doctor has prescribed. You should contact the doctor if the current dose doesn't seem to help. With the help of the health care team, you can also look into other methods such as massage and relaxation to help with pain.

Resources

Cancer Information and Support

Federal Resources

For more resources:

See *National Organizations That Offer Cancer-Related Services* at http://www.cancer.gov. In the search box, type in the words "national organizations."

Or call 1-800-4-CANCER (1-800-422-6237) to seek more help.

■ National Cancer Institute
Provides current information on cancer prevention, screening, diagnosis, treatment, clinical trials, genetics, and supportive care.
Visit................http://www.cancer.gov

> Cancer Information Service
> Answers questions about cancer, clinical trials, and cancer-related services and helps users find information on the NCI website. Provides NCI printed materials.
> **Toll-free**.................. 1-800-4-CANCER (1-800-422-6237)
> **Visit**............................ http://www.cancer.gov/aboutnci/cis
> **Chat online** .... Click on "LiveHelp" online chat from the home page.

■ Administration on Aging
Provides information, assistance, individual counseling, organization of support groups, caregiver training, respite care, and supplemental services.
Phone...............1-202-619-0724
Visit.................http://www.aoa.gov

■ Centers for Medicare and Medicaid Services
Provides information for consumers about patient rights, prescription drugs, and health insurance issues, including Medicare and Medicaid.
Toll-free.........1-800-MEDICARE (1-800-633-4227)
Visit..................http://www.medicare.gov (for Medicare information) or
http://www.cms.hhs.gov (other information)

■ Equal Employment Opportunity Commission
Provides fact sheets about job discrimination, protections under the Americans With Disabilities Act, and employer responsibilities. Coordinates investigations of employment discrimination.
Toll-free.........1-800-669-4000
TTY....................1-800-669-6820
Visit.................http://www.eeoc.gov

■ National Association of Area Agencies on Aging
Eldercare Locator

The Eldercare Locator is a nationwide directory assistance service designed to help older persons and caregivers find local resources for support. Areas of support include transportation, meals, home care, housing alternatives, legal issues, and social activities.

Toll-free.........1-800-677-1116
Visit.................http://www.eldercare.gov

■ U.S. Department of Labor
Office of Disability Employment Policy

Provides fact sheets on a variety of disability issues, including discrimination, workplace accommodation, and legal rights.

Toll-free.........1-866-ODEP-DOL (1-866-633-7365)
TTY...................1-877-889-5627
Visit.................http://www.dol.gov/odep

NonProfit Organizations

■ Aging With Dignity

Provides information and materials regarding advance directives. You can order the document Five Wishes, which states your end of life decisions for your health care team, and friends and family members.

Toll-free.........1-888-5WISHES (1-888-594-7437)
Visit.................http://www.agingwithdignity.org

■ American Cancer Society (ACS)

Mission is to end cancer as a major health problem through prevention, saving lives, and relieving suffering. ACS works toward these goals through research, education, advocacy, and service. The organization's National Cancer Information Center answers questions 24 hours a day, 7 days a week.

Toll-free.........1-800-ACS-2345 (1-800-227-2345)
TTY...................1-866-228-4327
Visit.................http://www.cancer.org

■ American Pain Foundation

Serves people with pain through information, advocacy, and support; pain and resource information, practical help and publications are available through toll-free telephone service and website.

Toll-free.........1-888-615-PAIN (1-888-615-7246)
Visit.................http://www.painfoundation.org

■ CancerCare

Offers free support, information, financial assistance, and practical help to people with cancer and their loved ones.

Toll-free.........1-800-813-HOPE (1-800-813-4673)

Visit.................http://www.cancercare.org

■ Cancer Support Community

The CSC is dedicated to providing support, education, and hope to people affected by cancer.

Phone: 1-888-793-9355

Visit: ....http://www.cancersupportcommunity.org

■ Center to Advance Palliative Care

Goal is to increase the availability of quality palliative care services for people facing serious illness. Offers training and assistance to health care professionals.

Phone.............1-212-201-2670

Visit.................www.capc.org

For patients and
families..........http://www.getpalliativecare.org

■ Family Caregiver Alliance

Family Caregiver Alliance addresses the needs of families and friends who provide long-term care at home.

Toll-free.........1-800-445-8106

Visit.................http://www.caregiver.org

■ Lance Armstrong Foundation

The Lance Armstrong Foundation seeks to inspire and empower people living with, through, and beyond cancer to live strong. It provides education, advocacy, and public health and research programs.

Phone.............1-512-236-8820 (general number)

Toll-free.........1-866-235-7205 (LIVESTRONG SurvivorCare program)

Visit.................http://www.livestrong.org

■ National Hospice and Palliative Care Organization (NHPCO)

Has information on hospice care, local hospice programs, advance directives in different states, and finding a local health care provider. It offers education and materials on palliative and end-of-life issues through its Caring Connections program, as well as links to other organizations and resources.

Toll-free.........1-800-658-8898

Visit.................http://www.nhpco.org

Caring Connections

Toll-free.........1-800-658-8898

Visit.................http://www.caringinfo.org

■ NeedyMeds

Lists medicine assistance programs available from drug companies.
NOTE: Usually patients cannot apply directly to these programs. Ask your doctor, nurse, or social worker to contact them.
Visit.................http://www.needymeds.com

■ National Coalition for Cancer Survivorship (NCCS)

Gives out information on cancer support, employment, financial and legal issues, advocacy, and related issues.
Toll-free.........1-877-NCCS-YES (1-877-622-7937)
Visit.................http://www.canceradvocacy.org

■ National Family Caregivers Association (NFCA)

NFCA provides information, education, support, public awareness, and advocacy for caregivers.
Toll-free.........1-800-896-3650
Visit.................http://www.nfcacares.org

■ Patient Advocate Foundation

Offers education, legal counseling, and referrals concerning managed care, insurance, financial issues, job discrimination, and debt crisis matters.
Toll-free.........1-800-532-5274
Visit.................http://www.patientadvocate.org